ONE PAN
PESCATARIAN

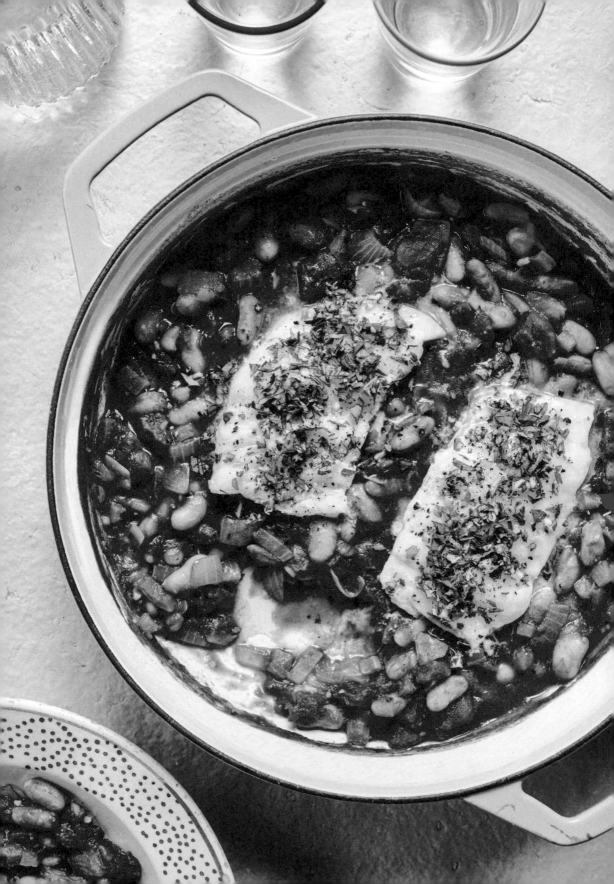

ONE PAN PESCATARIAN

100 Delicious Dinners – Veggie, Vegan, Fish

Rachel Phipps

First published in Great Britain in 2020 by Yellow Kite
An imprint of Hodder & Stoughton
An Hachette UK company

1

Copyright © Rachel Phipps 2020
Photography copyright © Haarala Hamilton @ Hodder & Stoughton 2020
Food photography on page 7 © Rachel Phipps

A CIP catalogue record for this title is available from the British Library

Hardback ISBN 978 1 529 34514 8
eBook ISBN 978 1 529 34663 3

Colour origination by Altaimage
Printed in Germany by Firmengruppe APPL

Hodder & Stoughton policy is to use papers that are natural, renewable and recyclable products and
made from wood grown in sustainable forests. The logging and manufacturing processes are expected to
conform to the environmental regulations of the country of origin.

Yellow Kite
Hodder & Stoughton Ltd
Carmelite House
50 Victoria Embankment
London EC4Y 0DZ

www.yellowkitebooks.co.uk
www.hodder.co.uk

Editorial Director: Lauren Whelan
Project Editor: Amy McWalters
Copy Editor: Clare Sayer
Art Director and Design: Nikki Dupin/nic&lou
Photographers: Liz and Max Haarala Hamilton
Home Economists: Rachel Phipps, Octavia Squire, Lara Luck
Props Stylist: Charlie Phillips
Production Manager: Diana Talyanina

CONTENTS

6   An introduction

7   A bit about this book
10 My pots and pans
14 Essential and unusual ingredients
18 A note on measurements
20 Mix and match meals

22 Vegetarian

92 Vegan

152 Fish

218 Index
223 Acknowledgements
224 About the author

An introduction

This is my elevator pitch. As a nation, we eat too much meat. We eat too much meat for it not to have a negative impact on the environment; too much for it not to have a negative impact on our health; and too much for it not to have a negative impact on our bank balance.

I am a meat eater and always have been. Apart, that is, from that time when I was a teenager and wouldn't eat red meat (except for sausages, bacon, my mum's delicious beef meatballs in tomato sauce and her spaghetti bolognese). I see now that my hang-ups at the time clearly had more to do with being put off by those horrible temperature-controlled trays of rubbery, well-done beef swimming in onions that I used to get at school, than actually disliking meat. Today I'm pretty sure I'll never cut meat entirely out of my diet. Skin-on, bone-in chicken thighs will forever remain my all-time favourite thing to make dinner with, and I think my life would become something less than it is now without an occasional big family roast, the table heavy with Yorkshire puddings and roast potatoes, a big joint of beef for Dad to carve, and a bottle of red wine to enjoy with all the people I love sitting around the table.

Most of the meat I cook and eat is for other people. My family is pretty much split into gender stereotypes. My mum and I prefer to eat a lot of veggies and fish, while the two boys think a meal is not a meal if they don't have a big hunk of meat somewhere on their plates. Okay, so I know a

lot of their protestations against plant-based eating are made to wind me up, but this did get me thinking; what are the barriers in place that stop people eating less meat, more fish, and more vegetarian and vegan meals at home?

While writing this book I've spoken to a lot of people – friends, family and total strangers – about their attitudes towards eating meat and the first thing I've learned is that plant-based meals (especially totally vegan ones) can feel intimidating.

Veganism, and the switch to plant-based diets, has exploded in popularity over the last couple of years, and I've had some fantastic vegan meals. I've also cooked some amazing recipes from vegan cookbooks and vegan food writers. However, I've found that a lot of vegan recipes are designed for, well, vegans and therefore suit a very different palate to the tastes of people who like to eat a lot of vegetarian and plant-based meals, but also love the taste of meat, poultry and game. Secondly, I know that a lot of the substitutions in vegan recipes that are there to replace things like eggs, dairy products and animal fats can put a lot of people off. With this in mind I've tried to make sure that the recipes in this book are the kind which – with the exception of my occasional use of tofu (which, as I do a lot of Asian cooking I see as more of an additional ingredient than a substitution anyway) – just happen to be vegan, rather than being made vegan by using substitutes or processed ingredients.

A bit about this book

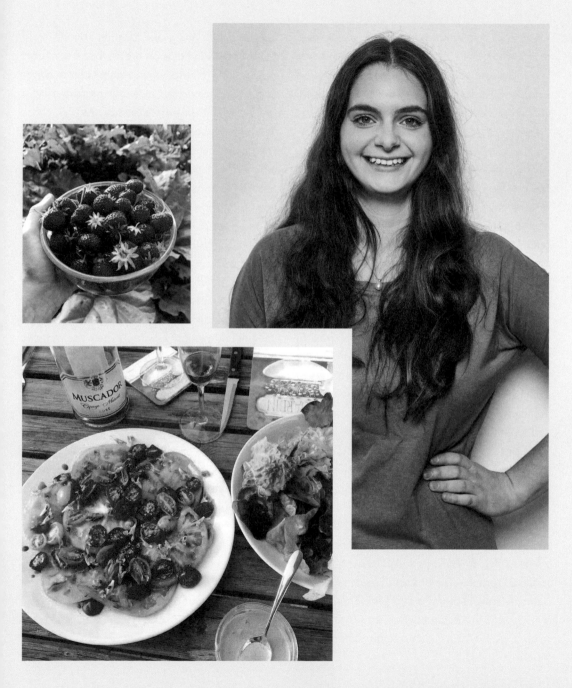

This is a book for meat eaters who are looking to incorporate more vegetarian, plant-based and fish-focused meals into their diets, but one that I hope will appeal to committed vegetarians, vegans and pescatarians, too.

Fish is a tricky one. When I started sending recipes from this book out to friends who were keen to test them I noticed that no one wanted to give any of the seafood recipes a go. I was not entirely sure why – possibly because fish can sometimes be quite expensive, and the difference between undercooked fish and something dry, rubbery and overdone can be just a matter of minutes. People often don't feel brave enough to cook anything past a couple of salmon fillets or a handful of frozen prawns at home. I think this is a sorry state of affairs. We live on an island, and yet we don't eat nearly enough of the fish that is caught off our shores. Tuna, cod, whitebait, salmon, mussels, mackerel, sea bass, sea bream, prawns, brown shrimp, scallops (or queenies, if your local catch comes from the Isle of Man), crab and squid are all native to our lakes, rivers and oceans, and I have included recipes for all of them in this book. Whenever you can, buy fish from sustainable British sources. I shop both in supermarkets, where I try to only buy fish that is clearly marked as such – the blue Marine Stewardship Council (MSC) label is a good thing to look for with regard to sustainability – and at my local fishmongers where I can ask questions about what I'm buying.

So why make this a one pan cookbook? Well, trying something new on a busy weeknight can be daunting. I literally write recipes for a living, and I still get nervous about trying something I've never made before on a Tuesday night when we're both hungry and tired, and just want a nice meal before deciding what to watch on Netflix. One pan recipes are easy; they tend to require nothing more than chopping, mixing, stirring, timing and sometimes a bit of marinating, and yield delicious results with little washing-up to do at the end. Consider the all-in-one nature of the recipes in this book as a sort of security blanket. My **Whole Roast Sea Bass with Fennel and Potatoes** (page 174), for example, is perfectly achievable for a special Friday night supper. When you're used to meat forming the backbone of every meal, doesn't the thought of tackling a roast fish, or plant-based supper, seem more manageable and less intimidating if you know the recipe is an all-in-one?

I'm not here to ask you to give up eating and buying meat (I'm certainly not going to); just to be more considerate to yourself and others when doing so. By doing your best to eat either a vegetarian or plant-based meal, or just something sustainable in the seafood department at least two or three times a week, you're already doing yourself and the environment a favour, as well as bringing down the cost of your weekly shop.

I know that most restaurants can both source better quality meat and cook it better than I ever could, so it is something I treat myself to when I'm eating out. I recently learned that the farming of grass-fed, organic cows incurs less carbon emissions than standard British cattle farming for many reasons, including the fact that they don't use pesticides. Although I already shop at an organic butcher's to supplement any supermarket meat, since discovering this I have been doing my best to choose organic milk, butter and yogurt too. If you're looking to lower your carbon footprint, cutting down on your meat consumption and buying organic dairy products where you can are good places to start.

I've split this book into three chapters: vegetarian, vegan and fish, so that if you've picked up a copy and are already following a specific diet you can easily find the recipes that best suit the way you like to eat and cook. However, I would still encourage you to dip into all the chapters. I eat meat, fish and dairy, and I'm the one who wrote this book, so naturally a lot of the recipes in here are up for a bit of chopping and changing. You'll find my **Kimchee Fried Rice** (page 76) in the vegetarian section because I like to add egg, but you can easily leave it out to make the dish vegan – I typically cook with vegan kimchee anyway (see my essential and unusual ingredients, page 14). The **Tomato and Root Veggie Casserole with Herby Dumplings** (page 96)

One pan recipes are easy; they tend to require nothing more than chopping, mixing, stirring, timing and sometimes a bit of marinating, and yield delicious results with little washing-up to do at the end.

– my favourite recipe in this book – is naturally vegan, but if you're happy to eat fish products, don't worry about finding vegetarian Worcestershire sauce, just use the bottle of the stuff you've already got lurking in your cupboard.

As a nation we need to change the way we eat, and restricting the amount of meat we include in our diets is a good place to start. I hope that the recipes in this book, will, at the very least, help you change some of the choices you make during the week, making it easier to incorporate more vegetarian, vegan and fish dishes into your diet.

My pots and pans

My kitchen equipment is a mad mix of battered, old and cheap (but still perfectly functional) pots and pans from my student days, and some rather fancy and utterly fantastic numbers I don't think I could currently afford if they had not been gifted to me in the hope that I'll mention them on social media along the way. Le Creuset, you utter heroes.

I use pots, pans, casserole dishes and roasting tins that have been both stupidly cheap and wedding-registry expensive, and I'm always happy with the results. While I won't pretend that fancy casserole dishes and baking trays are not nice to have, the quality of your cooking is very rarely impacted by how good your pan is. As long as it's strong, sturdy and the right one for the job, use what you already have and only buy what you think is good value for money. I'm also the kind of person who, when tackling a new recipe, just goes ahead and sees what will happen if I don't quite have the right tin or tray in my collection already, rather than going out to buy the specific item the recipe calls for. You should be that kind of person too, but be prepared for the fact that sometimes – but only sometimes – this might not work. You live and you learn, which is what cooking is all about.

I have listed all the pans that appear in my recipes, and the symbol for each is at the top of each one so you know what to use.

FRYING PANS

I have four of these: a cheap little 20cm (8in) one I use for small, quick, solo meals and for toasting things like nuts, and the rest are about 24–28cm (10in) that I use for bigger meals. Make sure you have at least one large pan with an ovenproof handle so you can stick the whole thing in the oven when making recipes like my **Asparagus and Goats' Curd Pancake** (page 57). I used to own a wok but an old housemate ruined it, and with a selection of good-quality pans I've not seen the need to replace it.

SAUCEPANS

All you really need in terms of saucepans is two different sizes: one really big one for making soups, sauces and stews, and a medium one big enough to cook enough pasta for 1–2 people or a smaller batch of something tasty. Both need lids, though if you already own saucepans without them, a flat baking tray perched on top will also do the job. Saucepans don't need to be expensive but make sure they have nice thick bottoms so that your food doesn't burn, and your onions don't brown too quickly.

SHEET PANS AND BAKING TRAYS

You will probably have at least a couple of these in varying sizes and quality, but I want to flag a couple of things that are important. First, you want nice, thick metal. Some of the cheaper, lighter trays will buckle in the heat of the oven and you'll get uneven cooking. Non-stick coatings are better, as they'll be less of a nightmare to scrub clean when you've roasted veggies on them. Also bear in mind that baking trays are not usually dishwasher friendly.

Next, you want to think about size. For dishes where only one or two elements are cooked in the oven, any size will do. However, you do want at least one tray that is as big as your oven can take for cooking entire meals for up to two people. If you crowd the pan too much things won't cook through, caramelise or crisp up properly. I have a pair of big square ones with very low lips around the edge for this, but for dishes with more sauce you'll want something with a higher lip so the juices don't run over the side.

CASSEROLE DISHES

These can be expensive but are immensely versatile. I use a big, round, shallow non-stick one with a lid to make curries, bakes, things like my **Spicy, Herby Two Pouch Mujadara** (page 108), and almost everything that benefits from being transferred to the oven afterwards or needs the lid put on at the end to help things cook. I also a have cheap cast iron pot that's just big enough to make a casserole for two. It's most often used in my kitchen for stewing things that are destined to be covered in fluffy dumplings like my **Tomato and Root Veggie Casserole with Herby Dumplings** (page 96).

OVENPROOF BAKING DISHES

Like most people, I have a random collection of different shapes and sizes of these. The ones I think are the most important to have are a big deep rectangle for pasta bakes like my **Spinach and Ricotta Stuffed Shells in Tomato Sauce** (page 50), and a round one that, at a pinch, can double as a pie dish. If, like me, you don't own a microwave, a little one is also useful for re-heating portions of food.

SLOW COOKER

There are so many different slow cookers out there so for your first one I'd recommend going cheap and cheerful until you see how much you use it. Important, though, is to get one of the 'sear and stew' models, where you can remove the metal insert to sear meat or soften onions on the hob before setting it, rather than having to dirty an extra pan for some recipes.

LOAF TINS

There are two standard sizes of these, a big 900g/2lb and a 450g/1lb one. You'll only need the smaller one for the recipes in this book, and I tend to halve most recipes I come across to fit in mine.

GRIDDLE PANS

You don't necessarily need one of these, but I own a big, flat, lined, non-stick griddle pan with a hot point at the bottom for setting over the hob for an indoor barbecue experience. Whenever I say that you can cook recipes designed for the barbecue indoors, this is what I use.

QUICHE/PIE DISHES

A simple but useful piece of kitchen equipment, and you don't need to spend money on anything special. Mine is glass, about 24cm (9½in) across, and only set me back £3.

BBQ

Barbecues come in all sorts of shapes and sizes with hugely varying prices. At my parents' house, my dad uses one of those smart rectangular ones; I have a cheap round one in my garden. Use whatever fits your budget.

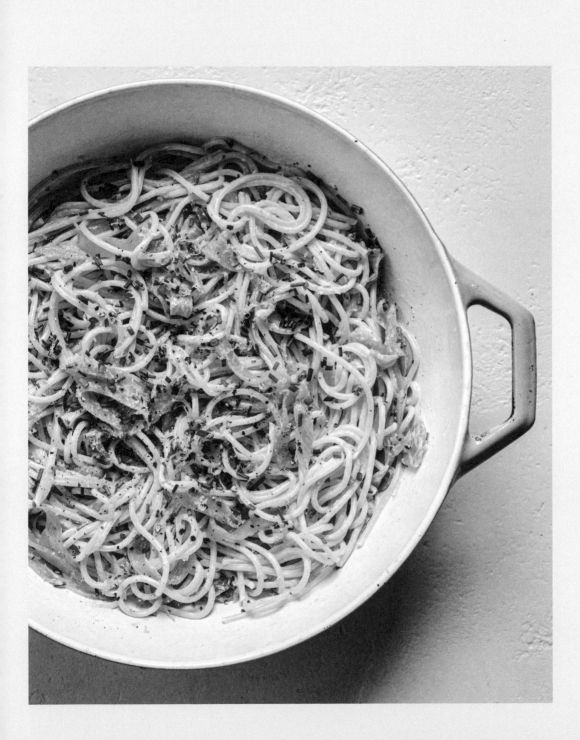

Essential and unusual ingredients

Most of the ingredients I've used in my recipes are common to every kitchen, but here is a bit more information about the slightly more unique ones that I love using and you'll find dotted throughout the book.

FRESHLY GROUND SALT AND BLACK PEPPER

I keep grinders loaded up with black peppercorns and English rock salt right by the stove where they are easy to reach, as well as on the kitchen table. I'm pretty sure I use them at every single meal, unless I'm making something of an Asian persuasion. If you're on a budget, or are a student, I've found that one of those pre-loaded salt and pepper grinders you find in the spice section of most supermarkets typically lasts an entire academic year. If you're choosing a grinder, the ones where you can select how fine the grind is are easier to cope with than having to mess around with how tight you've got the lid screwed on to control the grind.

SEA SALT

All sea salt is different. Every single brand from every part of the world tastes different and will have different sized flakes. I use *fleur de sel* from Guérande, harvested just off the Brittany coast, for almost everything; I love the flavour so much I can sometimes be found dampening my finger and dipping it right in the tub for a taste! Find a sea salt you like and stick with it; only then will you start to learn how big a pinch you need to balance out the flavours in your cooking.

LIGHT COOKING OIL

I'm not used to having room for loads of different cooking oils within reaching distance of where I cook. To combat this I keep just one big bottle of light olive oil for frying and roasting. It is so mildly flavoured I even use it in cakes and bakes that call for vegetable oil in place of butter. Choose an all-purpose oil that suits your budget and style of cooking: if you cook mainly Indian food, for example, vegetable or sunflower oil is the one for you, or if the wok is your weapon of choice, groundnut oil is also a fantastic all-rounder.

MILK

I don't drink it myself, but I grew up with a 2-pint carton of blue-topped full-fat milk sitting in the fridge door that I used in my baking, so I always used to specify full-fat milk in all my recipes. I still don't drink milk, but my boyfriend can't have a cup of tea or coffee without it, and he drinks semi-skimmed. And do you know what? Since I started using green top I have literally noticed no difference in my cakes, bakes and even panna cottas. So, unless I've specified otherwise, any dairy milk should work fine in all of these recipes.

GOLDEN CASTER SUGAR

I always list golden caster sugar and use it as standard both for health reasons (none of sugar's natural minerals have been stripped out by the refining process) and because I prefer the flavour it adds to cakes, bakes and sauces. However, if you prefer white caster sugar, none of the recipes in this book will be notably worse for it. I do still have white sugar in my countertop Kilner jar sometimes if I've bought a bag for making meringues or something similar where white actually is better. For a year, I lived in California where caster sugar is very difficult and expensive to find, so I just used granulated sugar for everything. Nothing went badly wrong because of the substitution, so you can be safe and happy in the knowledge that your tomato sauce won't taste overly sweet and sickly because you've grabbed the granulated instead of the golden.

KIMCHEE

This fermented mixture of salted and pickled vegetables is a staple of the Korean diet. I adore it and find ways of putting it in and on everything – it is particularly good spooned on top of a piece of avocado toast. While some supermarkets have started selling it in the Asian ingredients section, as it is a ferment, fresh really is best. You can usually find big tubs of fresh kimchee in the chilled section of Asian supermarkets, but I prefer to buy Kim Kong Kimchi (kimkongkimchi.com), which is made in North London, and can be found in independent delis, grocers and Whole Foods stores across London and the south of England. It's naturally vegan so keep an eye on ingredient lists if this is important to you as many traditional Korean recipes for kimchee often include added dried shrimp or fish sauce.

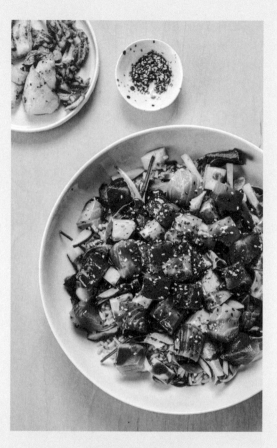

GOCHUJANG

Gochujang is a thick, slightly sweet, fermented chilli paste made from a barley, glutinous rice and soybean paste that is almost as common in Korean cuisine as kimchee, and a solid staple in my kitchen. You can find it online or in Asian supermarkets. Go for a Korean brand as I've not yet found a supermarket own-brand version that tastes as good or has the right flavour and consistency.

GOCHUGARU

Gochugaru are Korean chilli flakes, commonly used to make kimchee. They mostly come in tall, cylindrical canisters with a red lid, and you can usually find them in Asian supermarkets – failing that, you can always order some from Amazon.

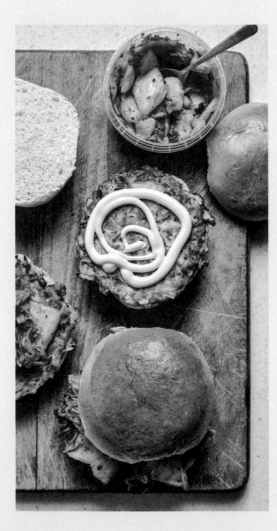

FURIKAKE

Furikake is a Japanese seasoning that is typically a mix of dried fish, dried nori seaweed, sesame seeds, sugar, salt and MSG, but I have never found two brands that are the same. Experiment to find a brand you like; I buy Sanchi, which is a simple, vegan-friendly blend of black and white sesame seeds, dried red shisho leaves and nori. You can usually find furikake in Asian supermarkets and health food stores that specialise in Japanese ingredients, and it is easy to find online. However, feel free to swap it for toasted black sesame seeds wherever you see furikake in a recipe.

KEWPIE MAYONNAISE

I rarely keep regular mayonnaise in my fridge; instead I keep Kewpie, a Japanese brand of mayonnaise that comes in a red-topped, soft squeezy bottle which you can now find in the Asian section of some of the bigger supermarkets (if you can't find it in the aisles try the sushi counter), Asian supermarkets and, of course, online. It's a little different to what we're used to, made with just egg yolks (rather than the whole egg), rice wine vinegar instead of industrial distilled, and (ironically, as I go to efforts to buy my furikake without it) added MSG, which makes it just slightly addictive in flavour. There has been a lot written about MSG, which is a common ingredient in Asian cooking. There is a strong argument that all the bad press it received is rooted in a historical suspicion of unfamiliar cuisines, rather than having a sound nutritional basis. Personally, I prefer my food as additive-free as possible, so long as it does not compromise on flavour. Kewpie mayonnaise is one of those instances where, as it is so delicious and such a versatile ingredient, I'd eat it regardless of what was in it. Life is all about balance, after all.

SOY SAUCE

When soy sauce is called for, I always mean dark soy sauce. If you do a lot of Chinese cooking there are two main types: light and dark, and both are common to UK supermarkets. Light is much saltier, and dark much more versatile and transferable across different soy-heavy cuisines. Japan has a few more varieties but go for the standard one, sometimes marked as koikuchi. Korean soy sauces are quite tricky to get hold of in the UK so I just use whatever I have to hand in all of my Korean recipes.

ALEPPO CHILLI

Aleppo chilli, sometimes known as pul biber, is my go-to if I want to add a chilli flavour rather than heat to a dish. I find regular dried chilli flakes can be a bit too full-on most of the time. Aleppo chilli is deep and warming, but still mild enough to sprinkle over salads, brilliant white slabs of baked feta and my morning avocado toast. It used to be tricky to find, but now it's readily available in the world ingredients section of most supermarkets.

MOLASSES

I use two types of molasses in my cooking: pomegranate molasses, which is tangy and fruity, and date molasses, which is dark and sultry. I think Odysea make the best supermarket examples of both, but you can usually also find them in most Middle Eastern stores. I'm particularly partial to drizzling pomegranate molasses – along with a handful of pomegranate seeds if I've got them – over a piece of toast spread thickly with hummus for breakfast or a mid-afternoon pick-me-up.

WHITE BALSAMIC VINEGAR

Think of this as a slightly tarter, more complex white wine vinegar and you're almost there. If you can't find any, it is probably called 'white condiment' or something similar on the supermarket shelves due to restrictions imposed by the Consorzio Tutela Aceto Balsamico di Modena. Because (of course) Italy has its own governing body for regulating balsamic vinegar.

A note on measurements

Everyone measures things differently so I have explained how I do it to give you the best chance of success when you're following these recipes.

WEIGHING SCALES

I have used my £15 Salter electric kitchen scales for measuring almost everything for as long as I can remember; I suggest you do the same for your cooking and baking. I believe these provide the best value in terms of accuracy and ease.

MEASURING JUG

I own a couple of measuring jugs marked up for liquids, but to be honest I never have the right one clean for whatever I want to measure (I've only got one of those slimline dishwashers) so I tend to use whichever one is on hand to pour water from the tap, or for all other liquids straight from their bottles into whatever receptacle I have to hand set on the fluid setting of my electric scales.

MEASURING SPOONS

All measurements listed in spoons are for level spoons unless I have stated otherwise. To make your life easier I would suggest avoiding artsy spoons joined together with an irritating key ring, in favour of a sensible plastic set that holds together with a magnet in the middle.

If, like me, the thing you want is never clean when you need it, learning that there are 3 teaspoons in 1 tablespoon will help prevent the need to pull on the washing-up gloves!

HANDFULS

I'm petite and have naturally small hands. This is worth keeping in mind whenever I talk about handfuls. Where I think my slightly smaller handfuls will truly impact the recipe, I've tried to provide a gram measurement instead.

GLUGS, SPLASHES AND DRIZZLES

Again, I've tried to give exact measurements whenever I think they will ultimately impact the recipe, but my glugs tend to be just over 1 tablespoon when I'm measuring oil and twice that for wine, and my splashes tend to be half the size of my glugs. I drizzle as thinly and quickly as I can for sparse effect – you can always add more, but once you've drizzled something all over a dish, it is almost impossible to take it away again.

SEASONINGS

When seasoning food over time you'll learn how much salt is in one of your pinches and how much pepper comes out of your grinder at once. But it is worth keeping the following in mind when following these recipes: my hands are small; that everyone seasons their food differently; and that my pepper grinder is always set on the setting that yields the largest flecks from the peppercorn. If your grinder does not have a special adjustment, loosening the screw at the top where you take the lid off to refill it will have the same effect.

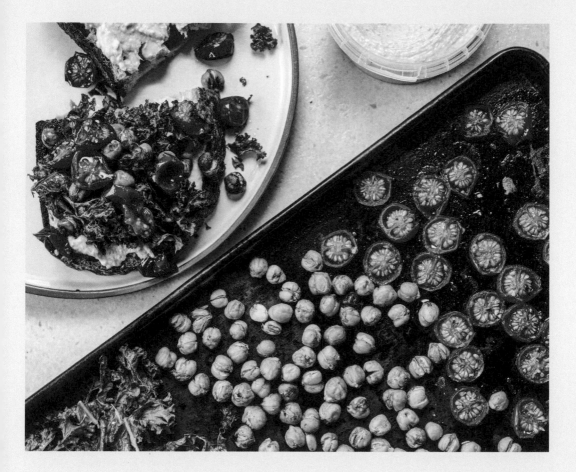

SCALING RECIPES UP OR DOWN

I'm rarely ever cooking for more than four people at once, and I'm most often just putting together solo lunches and suppers for the two of us at home. In many of the recipes in this book I've made notes as to which ones are particularly well suited to being scaled up or down, but as a general rule, if I've specified a certain type of baking tray or cooking dish, you might need to have two going in the oven at once if you've got a larger family to feed so as not to overcrowd the pan. If you are feeding a crowd and want to try a couple of the one pot, one pan dishes from this book at the same time, I've included some mix-and-match menu ideas over the page made up of dishes that go particularly well together.

Mix and match meals

While this book is designed as a collection of recipes that will help you easily produce entire, self-contained, one pan meals, life doesn't always work that way. Sometimes you want to bring more than a single dish to the table – when you've got friends over for dinner, for instance, or if you have a particularly big or fussy family – while still keeping the ease and convenience that one-pan eating offers.

Here are a few lists of recipes in this book that go particularly well together, some longer than others. When you're planning your menu do keep in mind not to double up on something like a certain cheese or on carbs, and to pay attention to differing oven temperatures and cooking times. Only you know what you, your oven and your kitchen can manage at once!

(V) = vegetarian, (Vg) = vegan, (F) = fish

menu 1

Kimchee Fried Rice (V), page 76

Spicy Korean Rice Cakes (Vg), page 146

Korean Salmon with Sesame Veggies (F), page 215

Spicy Cucumber and Silken Tofu Rice Noodles (Vg), page 148

menu 2

Warm Roasted Sprout Salad with Pecorino and Pear (V), page 30

Roasted Autumn Veg with Maple Mustard Dressing (Vg), page 102

Creamy Butternut Squash Risotto (V), page 60

Velvet Vegan Leek and Potato Soup (Vg), page 100

menu 3

Mexican Roasted Sweet Potato Salad with Honey Chipotle Dressing (Vg), page 28

Watermelon, Avocado and Feta Salad with Lime Dressing (V), page 68

Grilled Mexican Street Corn Salad (V), page 73

Plantain Tacos with Quick Pickled Onions and Smashed Avocado (Vg), page 122

Creamy Sweetcorn and Chipotle Soup (Vg), page 125

Sheet Pan Chickpea Fajitas (Vg), page 128

Crispy Cajun Coconut Prawn Tacos (F), page 183

menu 4

Tomato, Almond and Thyme Tart (V), page 35

Feta, Veggie and Lemon Bake (V), page 26

Tomato, Black Olive and Courgette Bread with Anchovy Butter (F), page 170

Mediterranean Salmon Parcels, (F), page 213

Orange and Rosemary Marinated Fish with Courgette Salad (F), page 207

Roasted Red Pepper, Spring Onion and Feta Frittata (V), page 48

Whole Roast Sea Bass with Fennel and Potatoes (F), page 174

Summer Veggie Crispy Gnocchi Bake (V), page 32

Baked Gnocchi with Tomatoes, Basil and Marinated Mozzarella (V), page 40

Tomato, Basil and Feta Orzotto (V), page 38

Gigantes Plaki with Feta (V), page 70

Veggie Paella (Vg), page 138

Easy Ratatouille Spiral (Vg), page 142

menu 5

Whole Baked Fish in a Sea Salt Crust, (F), page 178

Tomato Salad with Pomegranate Molasses (Vg), page 121

menu 6

Cheat's Chaat Salad (V), page 88

Cheat's Dhal Makhani (V), page 86

Dhal Baked Eggs with Chickpeas (V), page 90

menu 7

Deli Counter Hummus Pasta (V), page 117

California Kale, Orange, Almond and Mushroom Salad (Vg), page 112

Spaghetti with Muhammara Sauce (Vg), page 107

Spicy, Herby Two Pouch Mujadara (Vg), page 108

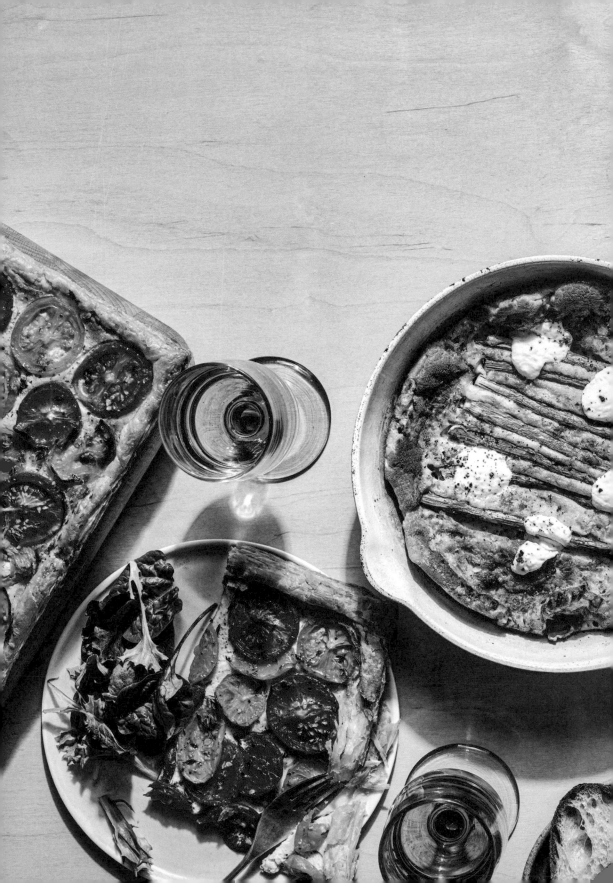

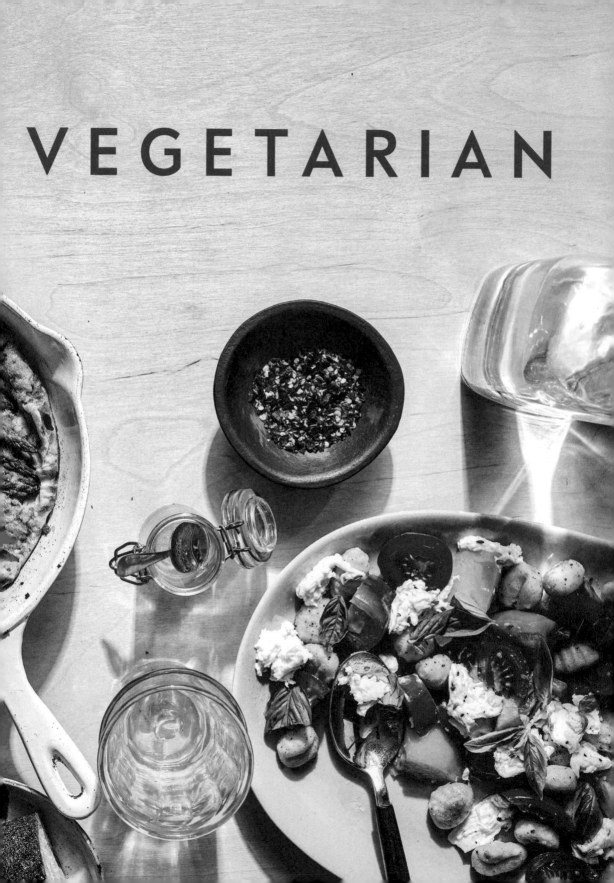

VEGETARIAN

These are what I like to call the gateway dishes in this book.

My natural default position when I'm cooking for myself is to go vegetarian, making something out of whatever pasta or grains I've got in the cupboard, bulked out with whatever I've got in my vegetable drawer and gussied up with a slick of butter or cream, a sprinkle of cheese or, most often, topped off with a baked, fried or poached egg with a runny, orange yolk

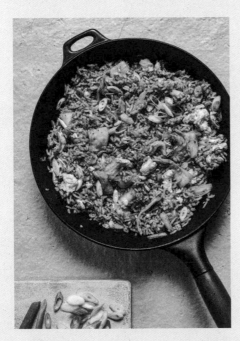

and the white just set. Regardless of how many dry goods are in my bottomless pantry, I've usually run out of fresh food when I've run out of eggs – I always buy a big box of twelve and we always get through them, a good eight or so usually on my account!

Kimchee Fried Rice (page 76) is my all-time favourite comfort food; I usually reach for the ingredients to make it whenever I'm home alone for the evening. My **Tomato, Almond and Thyme Tart** (page 35) with its unusual savoury, garlic frangipane is something I love to make for a slightly fancier than usual lunch in high summer, and my **Dhal Baked Eggs with Chickpeas** (page 90) is essentially a hug in a bowl on a cold, blustery night.

If you're used to including meat in every single meal, cutting it out while retaining eggs and dairy is a good place to start. As well as forming an essential source of protein (which, admittedly, can be a challenge to get right on an entirely meat-free diet) it is amazing what a little bit of dairy or a sunshine-yellow egg does to lift a meal.

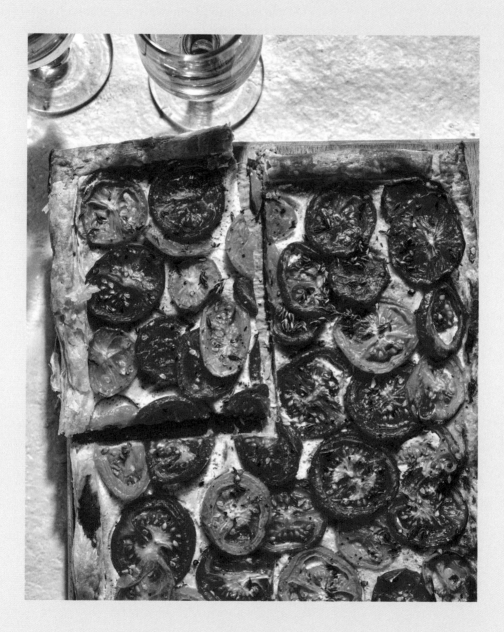

Feta, Veggie and Lemon Bake

SERVES 2

Preparation time: 10 minutes
Cooking time: 30 minutes

300g (10oz) mixed red, yellow
   and orange peppers
2 red onions
200g (1 cup) cherry tomatoes
½ lemon
2 tbsp extra virgin olive oil
200g (7oz) feta
1 tsp Aleppo chilli flakes
60g (⅓ cup) black olives
freshly ground sea salt and black
   pepper
small handful of fresh basil
   (*optional, for garnish*)

Feta cheese is beautiful when it is baked; it melts a bit like mozzarella and crisps up a little around the edges like halloumi, while somehow retaining some of its crumbly texture. It is simply delicious roasted with Mediterranean veggies, a little Aleppo chilli and lashings of extra virgin olive oil, served in big bowls with lots of crusty bread on hand to mop up all the cooking juices.

This dish is particularly good for using up the rest of a pack of feta you opened to crumble over a salad before it goes sour and any leftovers can also be warmed through and used as a base for scrambled eggs or my **Tex-Mex Tofu Scramble** (page 124).

1. Preheat the oven to 200°C/400°F/Gas 6. Deseed the peppers and cut them into rough chunks. Peel the onions and cut them into wedges and halve the cherry tomatoes. Halve the lemon into two quarters and cut them both into very thin slices.

2. Toss all the prepared vegetables and lemon slices together on a large baking tray with 1½ tablespoons of the olive oil and a generous amount of salt and pepper. Roast for 20 minutes.

3. Toss the roasting vegetables together so that they cook evenly, then crumble the feta in large chunks over the top. Sprinkle each chunk with the Aleppo chilli flakes and drizzle them with the remaining olive oil. Roast again for 10–15 minutes until the cheese has started to brown.

4. Roughly tear the basil leaves (if using) over the feta and vegetables and toss together just before serving.

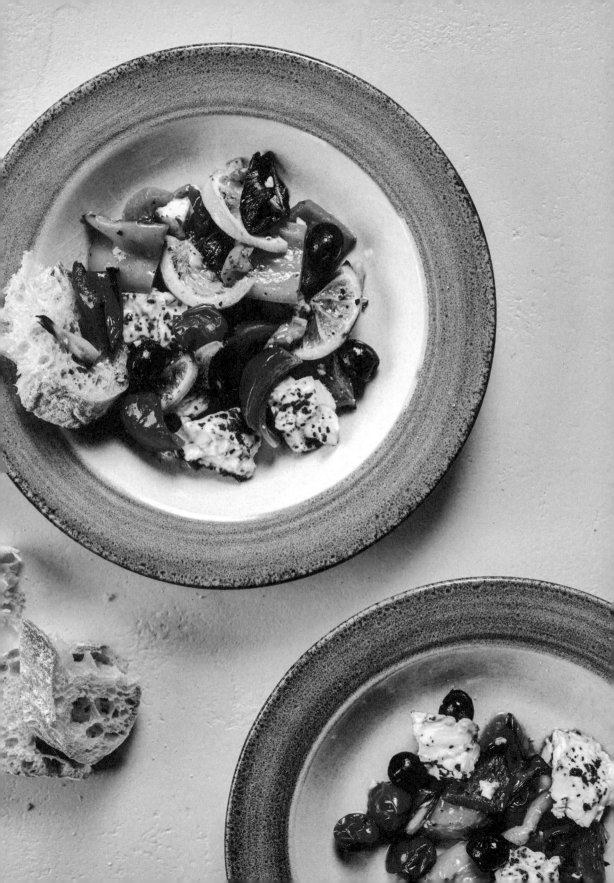

Mexican Roasted Sweet Potato Salad with Honey Chipotle Dressing

SERVES 1–2

Preparation time: 15 minutes
Cooking time: 20 minutes

For the salad
1 large sweet potato
½ tsp Cajun spice mix
1 tsp extra virgin olive oil
freshly ground sea salt and black
    pepper
1 small avocado
large handful of cherry tomatoes
120g (2 cups) tinned black beans
small handful of fresh coriander
large handful of rocket,
    watercress and spinach mix
small handful of pumpkin seeds

For the dressing
1 tsp chipotle paste
1 tsp extra virgin olive oil
1 tsp runny honey
juice of ½ lime

As a student I lived in Los Angeles for a year and, as well as an enviable tan from Fridays off spent down on Venice Beach, I came home with an enduring love for Mexican–Californian flavours. This roasted salad is full of contrasts: sweetness and spiciness from the honey chipotle dressing, creaminess from the cubed avocado, brightness from the cherry tomatoes, and crunch from a handful of pumpkin seeds added at the end. It's just the sort of thing I can imagine on the salad bar at my favourite SoCal grab-and-go lunch spot.

1. Preheat the oven to 200°C/400°F/Gas 6. Cube and toss the sweet potato (no need to peel it) with the Cajun spice mix, olive oil and a generous amount of freshly ground sea salt and black pepper on a medium sheet pan. Roast for 20 minutes until soft and slightly crispy in places.

2. While the sweet potato is roasting, make the dressing by whisking together the chipotle paste, olive oil, honey and lime juice. Peel and cube the avocado and halve the cherry tomatoes.

3. Remove the pan from the oven and add the black beans, coriander and salad mix. Pour over half the dressing and toss until everything is well coated.

4. Add the tomatoes and avocado, and drizzle over the rest of the dressing. Sprinkle over the pumpkin seeds before serving immediately.

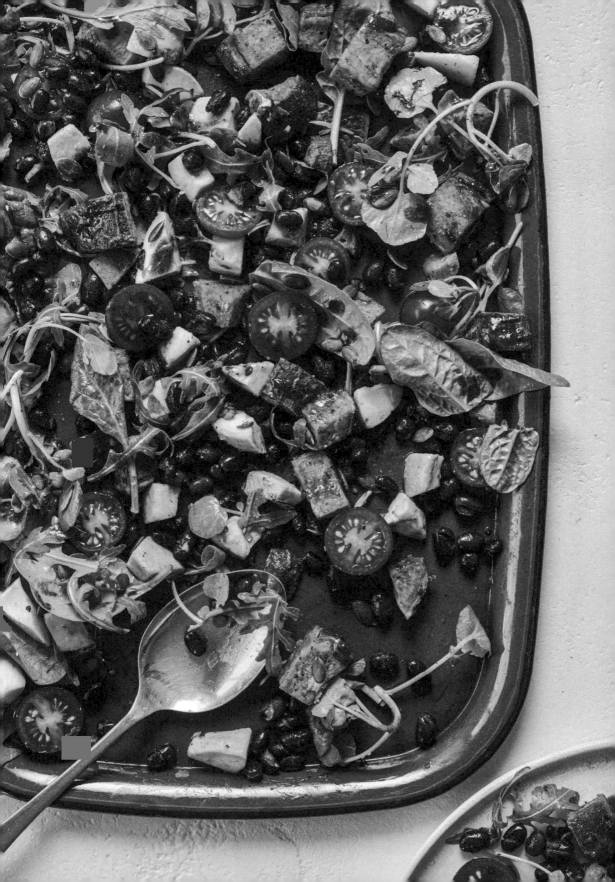

Warm Roasted Sprout Salad with Pecorino and Pear

SERVES 2

Preparation time: 5 minutes
Cooking time: 15 minutes

400g (14oz) Brussels sprouts
2 tbsp extra virgin olive oil
2 small pears
4 tsp lemon juice
2 tsp maple syrup
handful of pomegranate seeds
handful of pecorino shavings
   (*make sure you use a vegetarian
   version if this matters to you*)
freshly ground sea salt and black
   pepper

tip

*I use a vegetable peeler to
make my pecorino shavings, but
sometimes in Italian delis and in
Whole Foods you can buy a tub of
ready made shavings. If you can't
find pecorino, Parmesan would
make a good substitute.*

I like to make this in January when Brussels sprouts are at their best, and you can still get decent pears before the greengrocer displays are given over to imported Italian citrus and early bunches of wild garlic and asparagus. Please don't be tempted to make this salad any later than March, however, because while you can still buy Brussels sprouts then, I find these later varieties tend to be a lot more watery and don't roast up properly, reminding me of the boiled sprouts of those childhood Sunday roasts that I still can't stand. I learned this the hard way.

1. Preheat the oven to 200°C/400°F/Gas 6. Trim the dry base off from the Brussels sprouts (you won't need to do this if you're removing them from their stalk rather than just buying a bag of sprouts) and remove any darkened outer leaves. Take one half of the sprouts and cut them in half, then cut the rest into quarters to add a bit of texture.

2. Toss the Brussels sprouts together with 2 teaspoons of the olive oil and a generous amount of salt and pepper on a baking tray and roast in the oven for 15 minutes.

3. Meanwhile, core the pears and chop into bite-sized cubes (don't worry about peeling them). To make the dressing, whisk together the remaining olive oil, the lemon juice, maple syrup and a little salt, to taste.

4. Remove the Brussels sprouts from the oven and use a spatula to give them a good toss. Sprinkle over the pear pieces, pomegranate seeds and the pecorino shavings, then drizzle over the dressing. Give everything another toss, using the spatula to make sure everything is well coated in the dressing before serving.

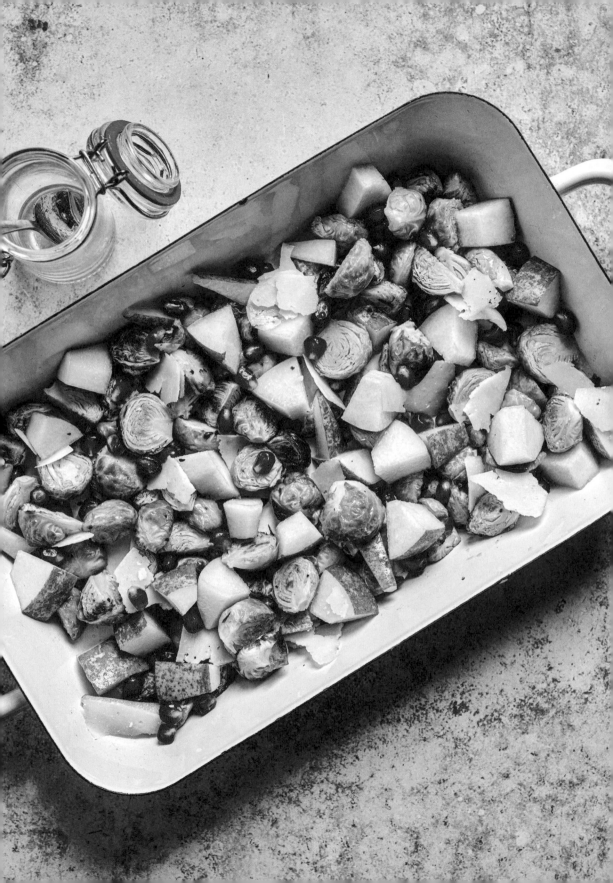

Summer Veggie Crispy Gnocchi Bake

SERVES 2

Preparation time: 10 minutes
Cooking time: 30 minutes

1 large red pepper
1 large yellow pepper
1 large orange pepper
2 large red onions
500g (1lb 2oz) pack gnocchi
1 tbsp olive oil
freshly ground sea salt and black
   pepper
handful of Parmesan or pecorino
   shavings (*make sure you use
   a vegetarian version if that
   matters to you*), for serving

It was a happy day in my kitchen when I discovered you could roast shop-bought potato gnocchi on a baking tray to incredible effect. I'd tried pan-frying homemade gnocchi before and it was a total disaster. In the oven the gnocchi goes magically crispy on the outside, but stays super-soft and fluffy on the inside. Buy flavoured gnocchi if you fancy something a little bit different; I'm a big fan of butternut squash and beetroot varieties.

1. Preheat the oven to 200°C/400°F/Gas 6.

2. Deseed all the peppers and cut them into bite-sized chunks. Peel and cut the onions into wedges.

3. Toss the peppers, onions and gnocchi together on a large sheet pan along with the olive oil and lots of freshly ground salt and pepper, making sure everything is well coated in the oil and that the onion wedges have broken up a little.

4. Roast the vegetable gnocchi mixture in the oven for 25–30 minutes, tossing halfway through, until the veggies are soft and slightly caramelised, and the gnocchi have started to go golden brown. Serve immediately with the Parmesan shavings sprinkled over the top, if using.

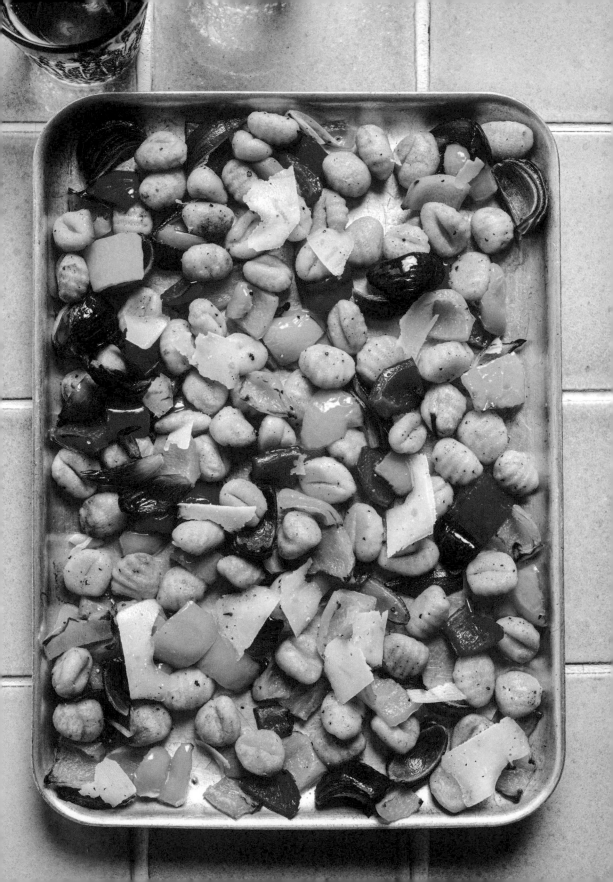

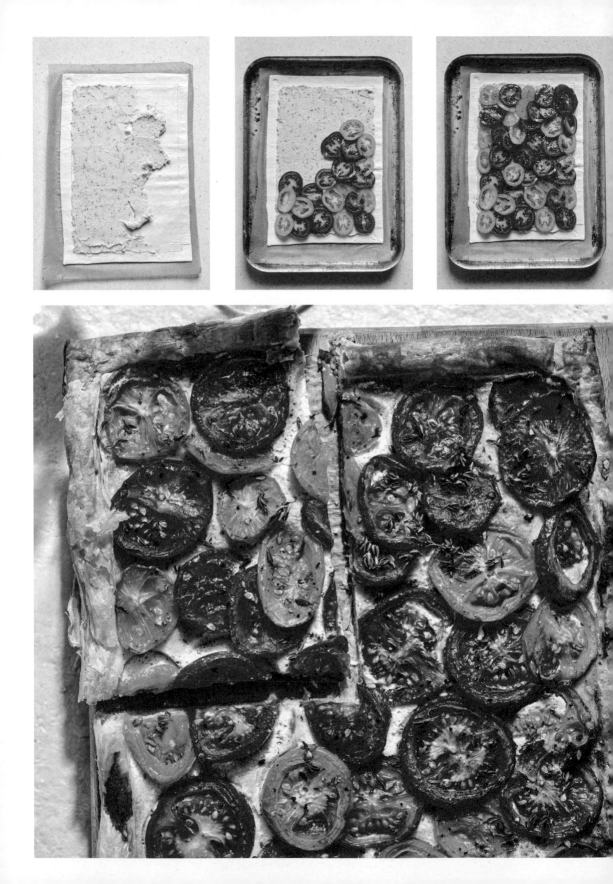

Tomato, Almond and Thyme Tart

SERVES 4

Preparation time: 15 minutes
Cooking time: 30 minutes

55g (4 tbps) unsalted butter, at
   room temperature
55g (½ cup) ground almonds
1 garlic clove
1 large egg
1 tbsp grated Parmesan (*make
   sure you use a vegetarian
   version if this matters to you*)
1 tbsp fresh thyme leaves
320g (11oz) sheet all-butter puff
   pastry
roughly 400g (14oz) mixed
   tomatoes
extra virgin olive oil
freshly ground sea salt and black
   pepper

tip

*If you have a basil plant or you've
got some leftover thyme, sprinkle
the leaves over the top to add
extra colour and aroma.*

Recipes for summery tomato tarts are ten a penny, but let me tell you why I love this one: the savoury garlic, Parmesan and thyme frangipane comes together in just moments and, after you've slathered it on a base of pre-rolled puff pastry, it is just a matter of covering it in ripe, rainbow tomato slices and baking it in the oven. I enjoy tackling long, multi-faceted weekend recipes as much as the next obsessive home cook, but this is all I want to eat at the end of a long summer's day. An ice-cold bottle of rosé to serve alongside it is not obligatory, but highly recommended!

1. Preheat the oven to 190°C/375°F/Gas 5.

2. To make the frangipane combine the butter, almonds, garlic, egg, Parmesan, thyme and a generous amount of salt and pepper in a food processor until smooth. If you don't have a food processor, crush the garlic, and beat everything together with a wooden spoon until smooth.

3. Line a sheet pan with baking paper and roll out the puff pastry sheet. With a sharp knife, score a roughly 2 cm (¾in) border around the edge, making sure not to cut through the pastry.

4. Using a spatula, evenly spread the almond frangipane to the edges of the border line.

5. Thinly slice the tomatoes, and arrange them over the frangipane. Drizzle with extra virgin olive oil, and finish with a good few grinds of salt and pepper.

6. Bake the tart for 30 minutes until the tomatoes are soft and slightly caramelised, and the pastry is golden.

7. Leave the tart to rest for 5 minutes before cutting into quarters.

Tomato and Courgette Baked Eggs

SERVES 1

Preparation time: 10 minutes
Cooking time: 40 minutes

2 courgettes
2 tbsp extra virgin olive oil
2 large garlic cloves
160g (¾ cup) cherry tomatoes, halved
small handful of fresh basil
2 large eggs
freshly ground sea salt and black pepper

tip

Fresh crusty bread to dip into those gloriously runny yolks is a must. If you have any basil left over, sprinkle it over the top of the pan before serving.

This is a simple vegetable dish using abundant, seasonal produce that I like to make when I'm cooking just for one. I first made it just after moving house, standing at the stove surrounded by boxes, using veg from the greengrocer's on the corner and a box of freshly laid eggs our French neighbour gave me when I went to say goodbye for the very last time. You can easily double the dish in the same size pan, but the courgettes will take a little longer to soften as you're crowding the pan a bit more.

1. Top and tail the courgettes. Halve them lengthways before slicing them into the finest half-moons you can manage.

2. Heat the olive oil in a shallow casserole dish or large lidded frying pan over a medium-high heat. When the oil is shimmering, add the courgette and a large pinch of sea salt.

3. Gently fry the courgette until it is soft and starting to fall apart. This should take about 15 minutes; if the courgette starts to brown at all, turn down the heat a little.

4. Crush the garlic and add it to the pan along with a generous amount of black pepper and fry until the garlic is soft and aromatic, another 5 minutes or so.

5. Add the tomatoes and cook for another 15 minutes until they are soft and starting to meld with the courgette mixture.

6. Turn the heat down to low. Stir in the basil, roughly chopped, and make two wells in the middle of the pan in which to crack the eggs. Do so, and put the lid on the pan, allowing the eggs to bake on the bottom and steam on top until their whites are just set. This takes 4–5 minutes on my hob, but don't worry if it takes a little longer on yours. Serve straight away.

Courgette, Lemon and Ricotta Fritters

SERVES 1–2

Preparation time: 10 minutes
Cooking time: 15 minutes

1 egg
190g (7oz) full-fat ricotta
zest of ½ lemon
generous grating of fresh nutmeg
100g (3½oz) courgette
½ tsp fresh thyme
4 tbsp plain flour
light oil, for frying
freshly ground sea salt and black
   pepper
tomato chilli chutney, to serve
handful of fresh salad leaves, per
   person, to serve

This is yet another dish born of a lunchtime fridge raid. I think I had a courgette left over from making the **Fried Courgettes on Toast** on page 47, and a bit of ricotta from making an Italian lemon and ricotta cake – our ricotta does not come in the same sized tubs as it does in Italy so I always find I have a little left over. These are great served alongside a green salad and a dab of tomato chilli chutney. Use your favourite; my mum makes a great homemade ripe tomato chutney and The English Provender Company also make a lovely one.

1.   In a small bowl, beat the egg and fold in the ricotta, lemon zest, a generous amount of salt and pepper and a good grating of fresh nutmeg – I'm not kidding when I say keep grating until you get bored and want to move on with the recipe – until just combined.

2.   Grate the courgette on the largest hole of your box grater and stir into the mixture. Fold in the fresh thyme and the flour, again until just combined.

3.   Heat just enough oil to cover the bottom of a large frying pan over a high heat. Once the oil is shimmering, fry heaped dessertspoons of the courgette mixture – flattening them with the back of the spoon as you go – for a few minutes on each side until very golden and just cooked through. Do this in batches so as not to crowd the pan, adding a little more oil as you go if you think they need it, turning the heat down a little if you think they're burning. Set the cooked fritters aside on a plate lined with kitchen paper to soak up any excess oil between batches. This should take a maximum of 15 minutes, depending on the size of your pan.

4.   Serve straight away with a good dollop of tomato chilli chutney and a some fresh salad leaves.

Tomato, Basil and Feta Orzotto

SERVES 2

Preparation time: 5 minutes
Cooking time: 25 minutes

large splash of light oil
1 small banana shallot
large pinch of sea salt
1 large garlic clove
300g (1⅓ cups) cherry tomatoes
230g (8oz) orzo
650ml (2¾ cups) hot vegetable stock
60g (2¼oz) feta
small handful of fresh basil

Orzo, the popular Greek pasta shaped like large grains of rice is such a pleasing thing. Depending on how you cook it, it can provide either a wonderfully textured base for a pasta salad, or a rich, sticky, almost risotto-like forkful when baked or simmered with a rich, flavourful broth. Here we're keeping things really simple with a comforting bowlful of orzo cooked, 'orzotto' style with fresh cherry tomatoes and vegetable stock, plus an added Greek twist of crumbled feta and roughly torn basil leaves to garnish.

1. Heat the oil in a medium saucepan over a medium heat. Peel and finely chop the shallot, and gently fry for 5 minutes or so with a large pinch of sea salt until the shallot is soft, but not quite starting to brown. Crush the garlic clove and add to the pan, frying for a further minute until fragrant.

2. Halve the cherry tomatoes and stir them into the shallots along with the orzo. Cook until the dry pasta is hot.

3. Add the stock, turn up the heat and bring the orzo to the boil. Then turn down the heat and allow to simmer for 20–25 minutes, stirring occasionally, until the liquid is all absorbed and the pasta is tender; it should have a risotto-type consistency.

4. Taste to see if more salt is needed before serving but remember, the feta will bring its own saltiness to the dish. Serve with the feta crumbled and the basil scattered on top.

White Peach, Mozzarella and Pea Shoot Bruschetta

SERVES 4

Preparation time: 10 minutes
Cooking time: 5 minutes

2 small garlic cloves
4 thick slices of crusty bread
extra virgin olive oil
2 large, ripe white peaches
2 x 125g (4½oz) mozzarella balls
4 handfuls of pea shoots
freshly ground sea salt and black
  pepper

This light, fruity bruschetta is my recreation of a dish I had at Polpo in Notting Hill years ago when it had just opened and you had to get there stupidly early to get a table. This is best made in the height of summer when peaches are in season. On the plus side, this means you'll probably have the barbecue going, so if you fancy this as a hearty starter rather than a light lunch, griddle the garlic bread straight over the coals, rather than in the pan.

1. Peel the garlic cloves and crush them lightly with the back of your knife. Rub each slice of bread with the garlic, then brush each generously with extra virgin olive oil. Heat a griddle pan over a high heat and toast the bread on both sides until browned.

2. Meanwhile, peel and roughly chop the peaches, and tear the mozzarella balls.

3. Pile the pea shoots on to the bruschetta toast, followed by the mozzarella and the peach chunks. Drizzle each generously with more olive oil and season well with salt and pepper before serving.

Baked Gnocchi with Tomatoes, Basil and Marinated Mozzarella

SERVES 1–2

Preparation time: 10 minutes
Cooking time: 20 minutes

250g (9oz) gnocchi
4 tsp extra virgin olive oil, plus
   extra for drizzling
2 x 125g (4½oz) mozzarella balls
zest of 1 small lemon
½ tsp fennel seeds
1 small garlic clove, crushed
1 tbsp white balsamic vinegar
300g (10oz) heirloom tomatoes
small handful of fresh basil
freshly ground sea salt and black
   pepper

In this simple but impressive salad, big chunks of heirloom tomatoes are scattered across the plate with torn pieces of fennel, lemon and garlic-marinated mozzarella. In an added twist, the dish is finished off with fresh basil, gnocchi made crisp and crunchy like croutons in a hot oven, and a good drizzle of your best extra virgin olive oil. Enjoy it on a weekend afternoon in the garden - it's equally as good as a solo treat as it is as part of a spread.

1. Preheat the oven to 200°C/400°F/Gas 6.

2. Tip the gnocchi into a roasting tray and toss together with 1 teaspoon of the olive oil and a generous amount of salt and pepper. Bake for 20 minutes until crisp and golden.

3. While the gnocchi is baking, marinate the mozzarella. Whisk together the lemon zest, fennel seeds – lightly crushed between your fingertips as you add them to the bowl – garlic clove, the vinegar, and the remaining 3 teaspoons olive oil with a large pinch of sea salt. Tear the mozzarella into bite-sized pieces and fold into the dressing

4. Cut the tomatoes into rough, bite-sized chunks. Scatter across a large serving plate, followed by the marinated mozzarella pieces, the basil, torn, and the crispy gnocchi, fresh out of the oven. Drizzle with olive oil, sprinkle with a little extra sea salt and serve.

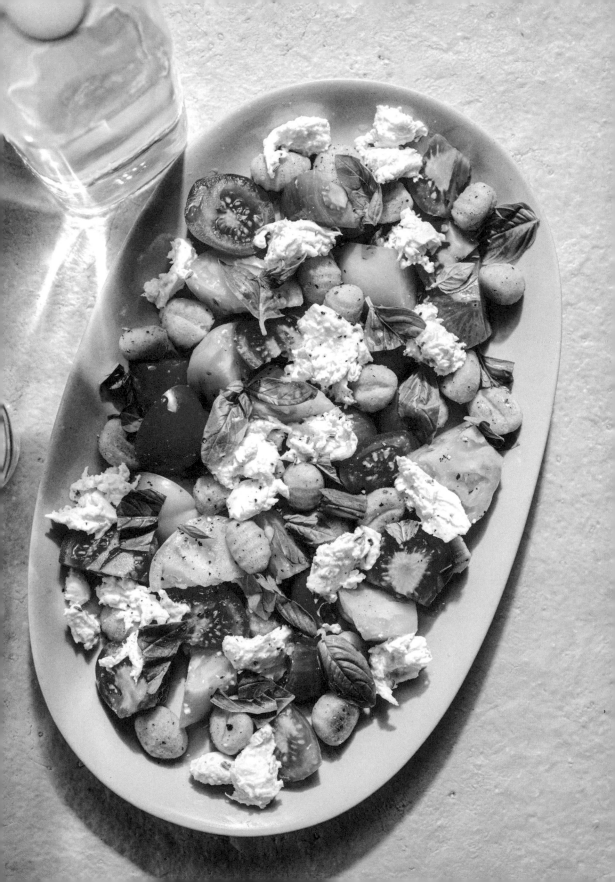

Feta, Muhammara and Charred Broccoli Ciabatta Sandwiches

SERVES 2

Preparation time: 15 minutes
Cooking time: 10 minutes

70g (2½oz) Tenderstem broccoli
1 tsp extra virgin olive oil
2 ciabatta rolls
½ batch of muhammara (below)
small handful of pomegranate
   seeds
40g (¼ cup) crumbled feta
small handful of fresh mint
freshly ground sea salt and black
   pepper

For the muhammara
160g (5oz) roasted red peppers
   (*from a jar*)
70g (½ cup) walnut pieces
½ tsp cumin seeds
½ tsp date molasses
juice of roughly ¼ lemon

Muhammara is a fantastic Middle Eastern dip made from roasted red peppers and walnuts, sometimes with fresh lemon added for brightness and some molasses to enhance the natural sweetness of the peppers. Here, it serves as a delicious spread in these moreish veggie sandwiches that I love to make out of leftovers for a working lunch on an early spring day. You'll only need half a batch however, so use the rest to make a portion of the **Spaghetti with Muhammara Sauce** on page 107.

1. Preheat the grill to high and the oven to 200°C/400°F/ Gas 6. Trim the broccoli and toss on a baking tray with the olive oil and a generous amount of salt and pepper. Grill for 10 minutes until slightly charred. Meanwhile, bake the ciabatta rolls for 8–10 minutes, or as per the packet instructions, until soft and warmed through.

2. Make the muhammara by blitzing the drained peppers, walnuts, cumin seeds, date molasses and a good pinch of sea salt in a blender or food processor until smooth. Season to taste with more sea salt and lemon juice.

3. To assemble the sandwiches, halve the ciabatta rolls and spread each generously with muhammara. On the bottom halves, divide the grilled broccoli, pomegranate seeds, crumbled feta and the mint leaves, either roughly chopped or torn. Top with the lids and eat immediately.

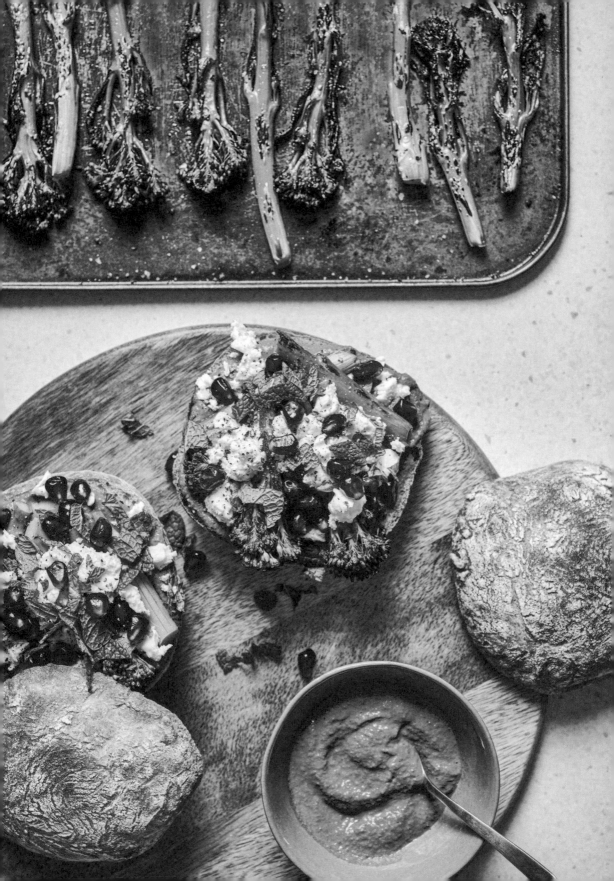

Turk-ish Baked Eggs

SERVES 1–2

Preparation time: 5 minutes
Cooking time: 15 minutes

unsalted butter, at room
   temperature
2–4 large eggs
60ml (¼ cup) double cream
a good pinch of cumin seeds
a good pinch of Aleppo chilli
   flakes
crumbled feta (*optional*)
freshly chopped coriander
   (*optional*)
freshly ground sea salt and black
   pepper

If I've not got anything planned for lunch and there are no old, repurposed takeaway containers of leftovers kicking around the fridge, I cook eggs. Sometimes I soft-boil them and use them as a dip for **Anchovy Butter** soldiers (page 170) and at other times I scramble them in a generous spoonful of coconut oil (it gives them a wonderful flavour and creaminess – give it a go!). If I've got a splash of double cream left (the supermarket never carries exactly the right size I need for a recipe) I make these rich, creamy, slightly Turkish-inspired baked eggs and arm myself with a stack of toast perfect for dipping, scooping and dunking.

1. Preheat the oven to 180°C/350°F/Gas 4.

2. Lightly butter an ovenproof dish and crack the eggs into it. Spoon over the cream and season well with salt, pepper, cumin seeds and Aleppo chilli flakes.

3. Bake in the oven for about 15 minutes until the whites are just set but the yolks are still lovely and runny.

4. Serve sprinkled with feta and a scattering of freshly chopped coriander, if using.

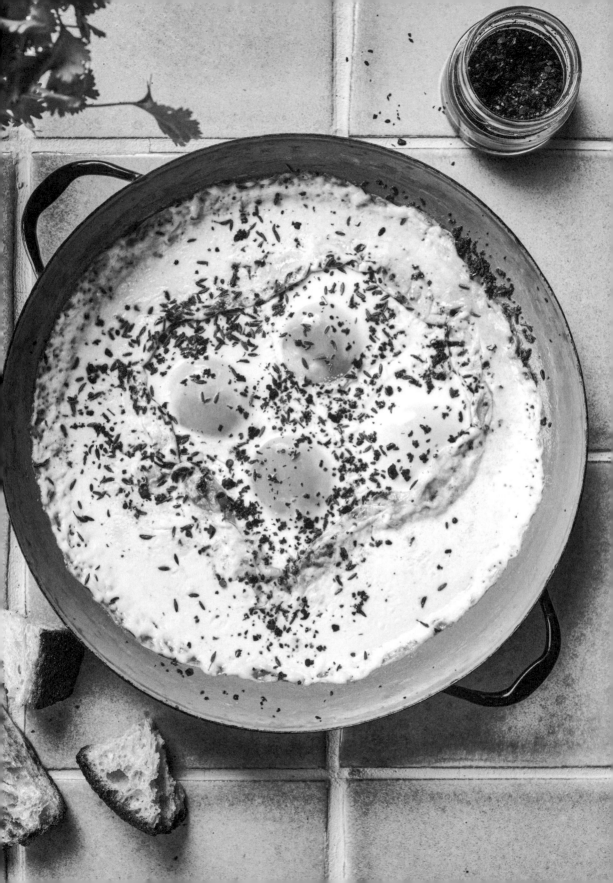

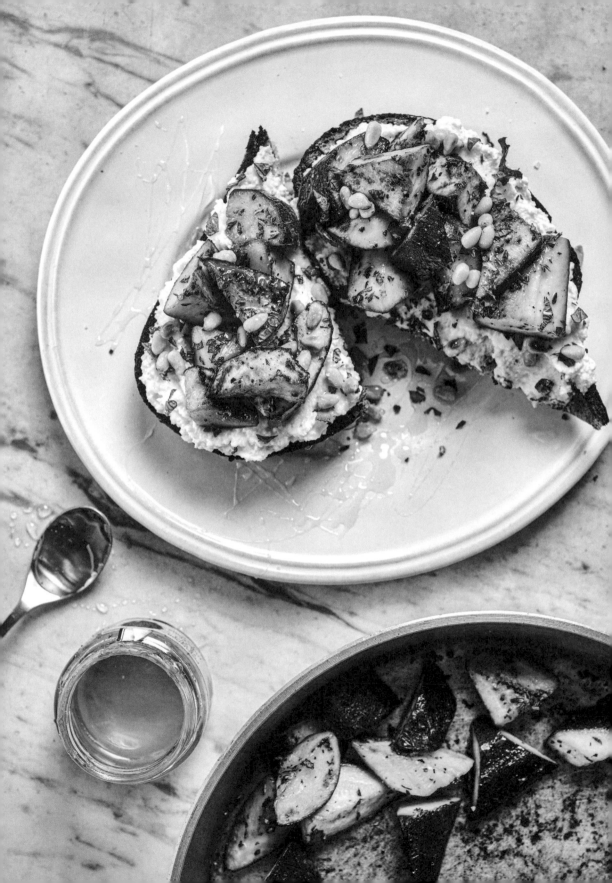

Fried Courgettes on Toast with Ricotta and Fresh Herbs

SERVES 2

Preparation time: 10 minutes
Cooking time: 10 minutes

20g (3 tbsp) pine nuts
2 tbsp extra virgin olive oil
2 small courgettes (about
  380g/13oz)
2 tsp white balsamic vinegar
2 tbsp chopped fresh mint
2 tsp chopped fresh thyme
2 thick slices of farmhouse bread
4–6 tbsp full-fat ricotta
2 tsp honey
freshly ground sea salt and black
  pepper

This particular recipe for something-on-toast is all about contrasts. Hot, soft, juicy courgettes cooked in just enough oil so that it just coats your mouth without being too fatty. Cool mint, earthy thyme, crunchy pine nuts, sweet, aromatic honey and sharp vinegar, all piled on to a slice of thick toast, crisp on the outside, but still soft and fluffy on the inside.

1. In a large frying pan over a medium heat, toast the pine nuts for 2–3 minutes until they start to turn golden. Set aside.

2. Heat the olive oil in the same pan over a high heat. Top, tail and roughly chop the courgettes into bite-sized chunks and fry in the oil along with a generous amount of salt and pepper for 6–7 minutes until the courgettes are just softened and golden on the outsides. (Tossing them around the pan only occasionally will help you get a nice level of caramelisation.) Stir in the vinegar along with half of the chopped herbs.

3. Toast the bread, then spread the ricotta over it and pile over the courgettes and the remaining herbs. Finish with a drizzle of honey and another few grinds of salt and pepper.

tip

I'm a bit of a truffle honey fiend, so if you love it as much as I do it would be delicious drizzled on top instead.

Roasted Red Pepper, Spring Onion and Feta Frittata

SERVES 4

Preparation time: 5 minutes
Cooking time: 50 minutes

300g (10oz) new potatoes
1 large red, yellow or orange
   pepper
1 tbsp extra virgin olive oil (*I
   sometimes use chilli oil for an
   added kick!*)
6 large eggs
3–4 large spring onions
70g (2½oz) feta
freshly ground sea salt and black
   pepper

When I used to have an office job I made a frittata most Sunday nights to use as breakfasts or lunches for the week. They were great for using up any odds and ends of vegetables and cheese that were still hanging around the fridge. It was a much healthier habit than indulging in the stupidly cheap breakfast wraps from the cafeteria stuffed with sausages, bacon and black pudding with the option of an extra egg or hash brown! Without my pre-made breakfast frittata they would have just been too tempting.

1. Preheat the oven to 200°C/400°F/Gas 6. Halve the new potatoes and core and deseed the pepper, cutting it into bite-sized chunks. Toss the veggies together with the olive oil and lots of salt and pepper in a square baking dish – mine is roughly 20cm (8in) square. Transfer to the oven to roast for 30 minutes.

2. Meanwhile, whisk together the eggs with another few grinds of salt and pepper until well combined. Set aside.

3. Remove the dish from the oven and toss the potatoes and the peppers around a bit to make sure they cook evenly. By now they should be just tender and starting to brown. Top, tail and slice the spring onions and sprinkle over the top. Crumble over the feta, then pour over the egg mixture.

4. Reduce the oven temperature to 180°C/350°F/Gas 4 and return the dish to the oven for 20 minutes. It should puff up well, sometimes crack slightly, and be golden brown on top. Leave it for 5 minutes or so to deflate before slicing. I like to serve this at room temperature.

Savoury Wild Mushroom Oatmeal

SERVES 1

Preparation time: 5 minutes
Cooking time: 5 minutes

10g (¼oz) dried wild mushrooms
knob of unsalted butter
1 large banana shallot
60g (2¼oz) mixed mushrooms
150ml (⅔ cup) milk
1 tsp red miso paste
45g (½ cup) porridge oats
freshly ground sea salt and black
  pepper
small handful of fresh flat leaf
  parsley
freshly grated Parmesan (*make
  sure you use a vegetarian
  version if this matters to you*)

I have a funny thing about porridge oats. For breakfast in England I can't stand anything creamy and oat-based, but in America as a student I'd have a bowl of oatmeal for breakfast every morning with maple syrup and blueberries. It turns out that the way to get me to like porridge oats this side of the pond is to make them savoury, flavouring them with miso, and topping them with a hearty mixture of wild mushrooms. I have this for lunch on very cold autumn days.

1. Soak the dried mushrooms in 150ml (⅔ cup) boiling water for 15 minutes. Set aside.

2. Heat the butter in a small lidded saucepan over a medium-high heat until frothy. Peel and finely chop the shallot and gently fry with a pinch of salt for about 5 minutes until soft.

3. Slice the mushrooms and add to the pan, raising the heat and cooking them for a further 5 minutes or so until they are soft and slightly browned and any excess water has bubbled away.

4. Drain the dried mushrooms, setting aside the soaking water. Roughly chop the mushrooms and add to the pan, cooking until heated through. Remove from the pan, and set aside.

5. Top the mushroom soaking liquid up to 150ml (⅔ cup) with milk and combine in the saucepan with the miso and oats. Bring to the boil, turning the heat right down the moment you see bubbles. Leave to simmer for 5 minutes, uncovered.

6. Remove the oats from the heat and put on the lid, leaving the oatmeal to steam for a further 5 minutes before stirring in another small knob of butter and the mushroom mixture.

7. Serve in warm bowls with chopped parsley and Parmesan.

Spinach and Ricotta Stuffed Shells in Tomato Sauce

SERVES 2–3

Preparation time: 30 minutes
Cooking time: 40 minutes (plus 10
 minutes resting time)

140g (5oz) giant pasta shells
 (conchiglioni)
200g (7oz) frozen spinach,
 defrosted
250g (1 cup) ricotta
20g (¾oz) Parmesan (*make sure
 you use a vegetarian version if
 this matters to you*), plus extra
 for topping
½ tsp sea salt
¼ tsp grated nutmeg
400ml (1⅔) cups passata
125ml (½ cup) vegetable stock
1 tsp golden caster sugar
small handful of fresh flat leaf
 parsley
1 garlic clove
50g (1 cup) fresh breadcrumbs
1 tsp extra virgin olive oil

I've always loved the look of a big, bubbling dish of baked pasta shells, filled with something creamy and delicious, sitting in a rich sauce and covered with melted cheese and crispy breadcrumbs. However, I find cooking a filling, making a sauce, and pre-cooking the giant pasta shells – the Italians call them conchiglioni – before having to assemble the whole thing a little too much for a busy weeknight. Not here.

All you need to do to produce this impressive-looking dish is to soak the shells in a bowl of boiling water while you mix together a few ingredients – no need to worry about pre-cooking anything. Once you've filled them, they nestle happily in the passata.

1. Preheat the oven to 180°C/350°F/Gas 4 and boil the kettle. Leave the pasta shells to soak in a bowl of boiling water for 20 minutes.

2. Meanwhile, squeeze any excess water out of the spinach over the kitchen sink before roughly chopping it and transferring it to a small bowl. Add the ricotta, Parmesan, sea salt and nutmeg and fold to combine.

3. Mix the passata, vegetable stock and sugar together in the bottom of a large baking dish and set aside.

4 Finely chop the parsley and the garlic clove then combine with the breadcrumbs and olive oil; again setting aside.

5. Drain the pasta shells and fill each one with a heaped

Continued overleaf...

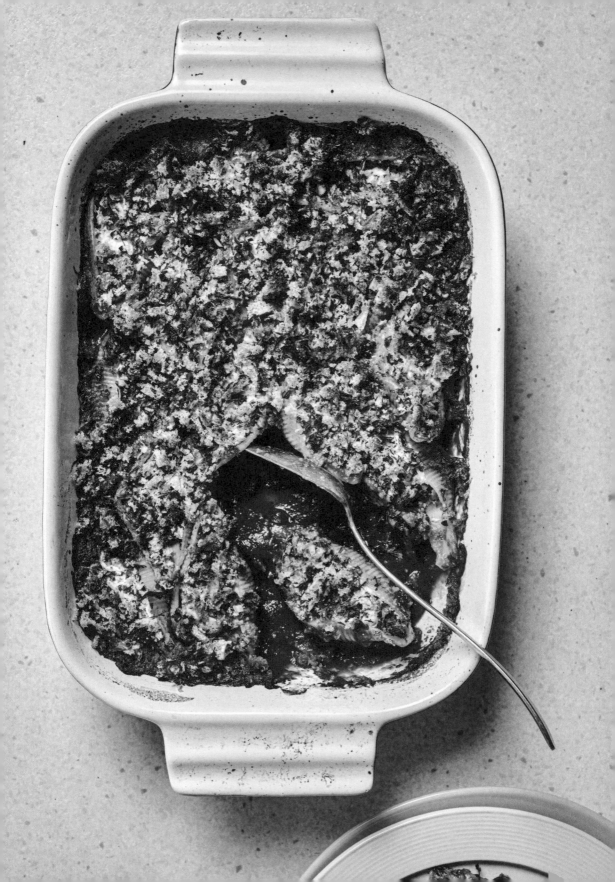

teaspoon of ricotta and spinach filling before nestling them in the tomato sauce. Once you've filled the entire dish (you may have a few extra shells – I've allowed for a few to accidentally split), sprinkle with the breadcrumb mixture and grate over a little extra Parmesan.

6. Bake in the oven for 40 minutes until the pasta is just tender, the sauce is bubbling and the breadcrumbs are golden. Allow to rest for 10 minutes before serving.

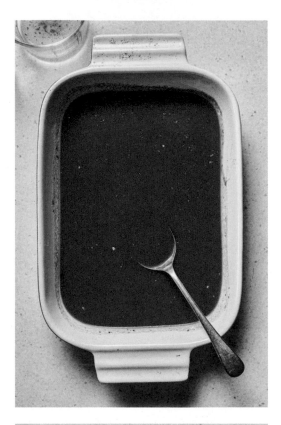

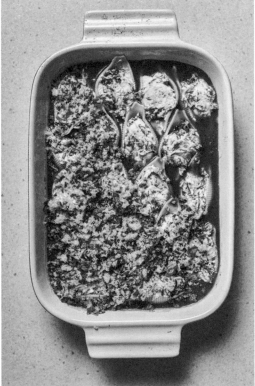

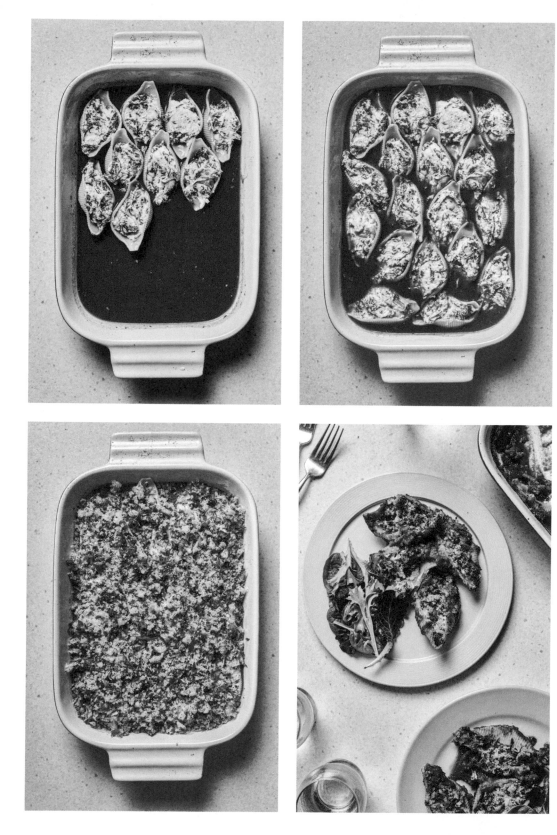

Spinach, Egg and Mushroom Dutch Baby Pancake

SERVES 1

Preparation time: 5 minutes
Cooking time: 50 minutes

3 large eggs

5½ tbsp milk

3 tbsp plain flour

50g (2oz) frozen spinach (about 2 frozen lumps), defrosted

unsalted butter, for frying

100g (3½oz) chestnut mushrooms

small handful of fresh flat leaf parsley

freshly grated Parmesan (*optional; make sure you use a vegetarian version if this matters to you*)

freshly ground sea salt and black pepper

Here it is – the perfect hearty vegetarian solo supper. This recipe started its life as a hybrid between a Dutch baby pancake and a traditional French ham, cheese and egg crêpe I created for *BBC Food*. The original featured ribbons of wafer-thin ham, but while I was perfecting the recipe I realised that it would actually taste so much better piled with buttery, parsley-flavoured mushrooms.

1. Preheat the oven to 200°C/400°F/Gas 6. Start by making the pancake batter. Whisk together 2 of the eggs, the milk, flour and a generous amount of both salt and pepper in a small jug or bowl.

2. Over the sink, squeeze as much of the water as you can out of the defrosted spinach, separating the leaves as much as you can. Gently stir the spinach into the pancake batter and set aside.

3. Next, prepare the mushrooms. Melt a knob of unsalted butter over a medium heat in a medium, non-stick frying pan with an ovenproof handle.

4. Slice the mushrooms, adding them to the pan along with another generous amount of salt and pepper. Gently fry them for a few minutes until they're soft and starting to go brown around the edges. Stir in the parsley, then remove the mushrooms from the pan and set aside.

5. Using a piece of kitchen paper, wipe out the pan and return it to a medium heat. Add another generous knob of butter. Allow it to melt completely, then swill the pan around, swishing the melted butter up the edges so that as much of the pan as possible is coated in melted butter.

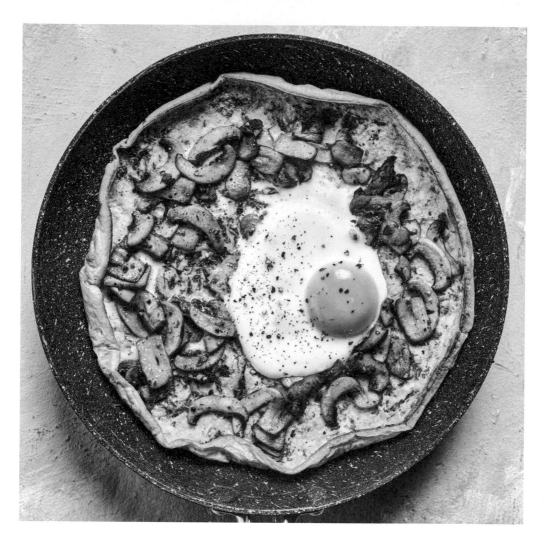

6. Give the batter a gentle stir, then pour it into the middle of the hot buttered pan before transferring immediately to the oven. Bake for 10 minutes – the pancake should set and start to puff up around the edges.

7. Sprinkle the cooked mushrooms over the pancake before cracking the remaining egg into the middle. Return the pancake to the oven for another 5 minutes until the egg white is set but the yolk is still runny.

8. Sprinkle the Parmesan over the top, if using, before sliding the pancake out of the pan on to a warm plate.

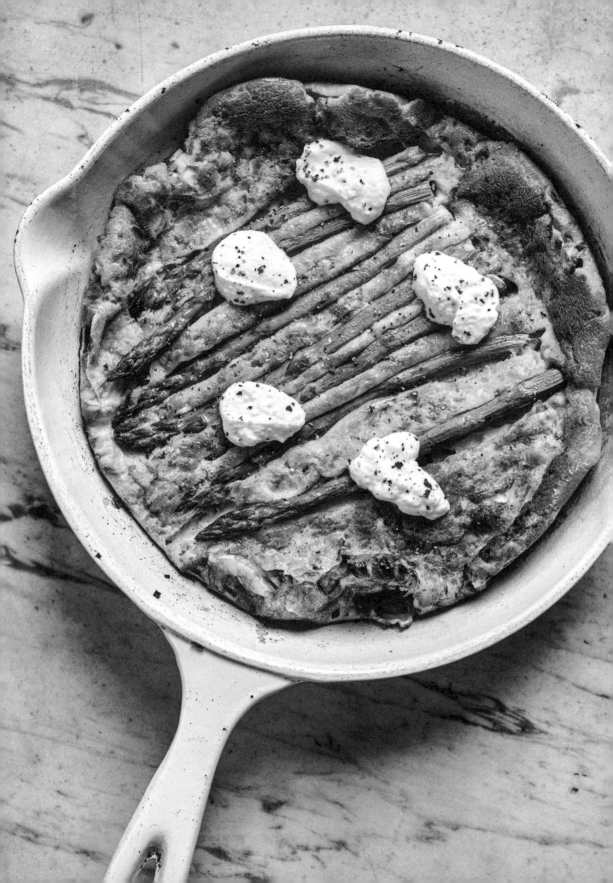

Asparagus and Goats' Curd Pancake

SERVES 1

Preparation time: 5 minutes
Cooking time: 20 minutes

2 large eggs
5½ tbsp milk
3 tbsp plain flour
unsalted butter, for frying
1 large banana shallot, finely
   chopped
100g (3½oz) asparagus
80g (3oz) goats' curd
freshly ground sea salt and black
   pepper

This dish is inspired by the Périgord region that follows the Dordogne River through south-west France, one of my favourite places to eat outside of Brittany. I adore its Périgord truffles and walnuts, Rocamadour goats' cheese and tiny, intensely perfumed gariguette strawberries, but this dish is a celebration of the region's wonderful asparagus, standing to attention at Sarlat's Saturday morning market. You should never do something too fussy with asparagus; a simple treatment like this pancake really shows it at its best. Beautiful stalks of English asparagus start to appear at the end of April, so this is the perfect dish for spring and early summer.

1. Preheat the oven to 200°C/400°F/Gas 6.

2. Whisk together the eggs, milk, flour and a generous amount of salt and pepper into a sticky batter. Set aside.

3. Place a medium-large non-stick frying pan over a medium heat. Add a large knob of butter; once it has melted and gone frothy add the shallot and a large pinch of salt, gently fry until the shallot has gone soft and just started to brown. This should take about 5 minutes.

4. Remove the pan from the heat and pour over the batter. Arrange the asparagus spears side by side like soldiers in the batter and transfer to the oven to bake for 15 minutes until the batter is set, the asparagus is tender and the edges of the pancake have gone all puffy and golden.

5. Scatter the goats' curd over the top of the pancake and serve immediately as it just starts to melt.

Cacio e Pepe Eggy Bread Crumpets

SERVES 2

Preparation time: 5 minutes
Cooking time: 5 minutes

2 large eggs
1 tbsp milk
4 tbsp freshly grated Parmesan
(*make sure you use a
vegetarian version, if this
matters to you*)
4 crumpets
generous splash of light oil
freshly ground sea salt and black
pepper
Heinz tomato ketchup, to serve

Eggy bread – always served with Heinz tomato ketchup – is a seriously big deal in my family. No Saturday or Sunday breakfast is better than when I come downstairs at my parents' house to find my dad standing over a pan of egg-soaked bread. We abandoned using sliced bread years ago; now our preference is to use stale slices of French stick. However, when I'm making breakfast just for me, I make my eggy bread with crumpets, letting the egg drip into the holes for the perfect mixture of crispiness, sponginess and egginess in each bite.

1. Whisk together the eggs, milk, Parmesan, a generous amount of sea salt and more freshly ground black pepper than you think you could possibly need until combined in a shallow dish.

2. Place the crumpets, hole side down, in the egg mixture and leave to soak for a minute or two, before turning over and soaking the other side.

3. Meanwhile, heat the oil over a medium-high heat in a (preferably non-stick) frying pan, large enough to accommodate all the crumpets.

4. Place the crumpets, flat side down on the pan and allow to gently fry for 2–3 minutes until the bottoms are crisp and golden. Meanwhile, divide the leftover egg mixture between the crumpets, gradually pouring it over them bit by bit, to allow the egg to soak into the holes.

5. Flip the crumpets quickly so the tops have the chance to turn golden and the egg inside the holes has a chance to set. Serve with a generous amount of ketchup in which to dip each bite.

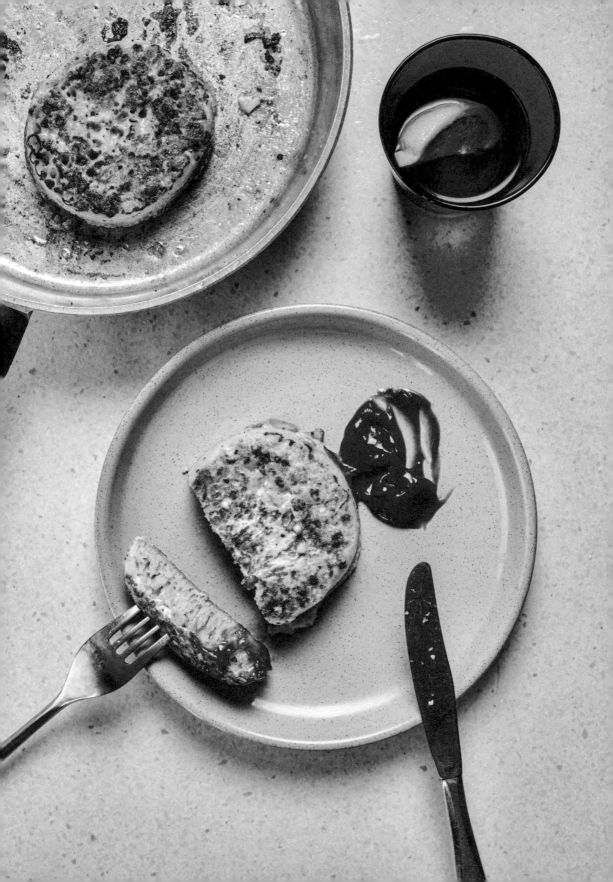

Creamy Butternut Squash Risotto

SERVES 2

Preparation time: 10 minutes
Cooking time: 1 hour

unsalted butter
1 small onion
150g (5oz) butternut squash,
   grated
100g (3½oz) butternut squash,
   cubed
150g (¾cup) risotto rice
100ml (6 tbsp) dry white wine
800ml (3⅓ cups) hot vegetable
   stock
15g (3 tbsp) Parmesan
   shavings (*make sure you use
   a vegetarian version if this
   matters to you*), plus extra to
   serve
½ tbsp fresh sage, chopped
sea salt and freshly ground black
   pepper

Every time I have butternut squash in the fridge this is the thing I want to make the most. It is basically one big – rather elegant – autumnal hug in a bowl.

If this is your first time making risotto, don't panic, it's really easy. Take cooking times with a pinch of salt and gradually add the stock until you're happy with the consistency. I've included measurements and timings here but, depending on how hot your hob is, and the size and thickness of your pan, you might need more or less stock than that. It's okay to add more if your rice still has a bit too much bite to it. Once you've made a couple of risottos, you'll know what works best.

1. Heat a knob of butter in a shallow casserole dish or large frying pan over a medium heat. Peel and finely chop the onion and gently fry it, along with a good pinch of sea salt, for roughly 5 minutes until it has softened and darkened in colour, but has not yet started to brown.

2. Add both the grated and cubed squash and cook for a further 15 minutes until the grated squash is tender and the cubes have started to soften.

3. Stir in the risotto rice and cook for another couple of minutes until the rice is hot.

4. Turn the heat down to medium-low. Stir in the white wine and allow to bubble away. Add a ladle of the hot stock and again allow it to bubble away, stirring every few minutes.

Continued overleaf...

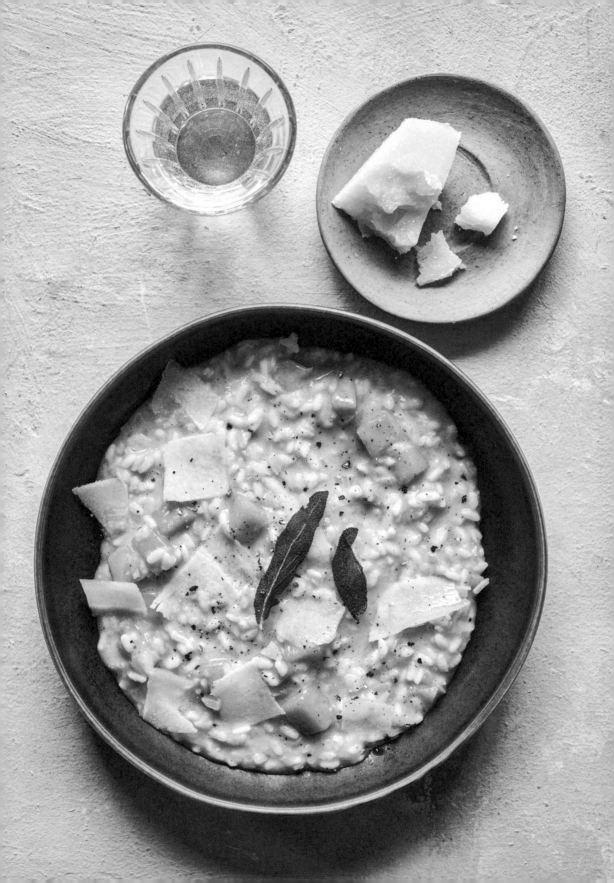

5. Keep going for 35–40 minutes until all the stock has been absorbed and the rice is tender.

6. Once you're happy with the texture of the rice, stir in the Parmesan and another small knob of butter, then season to taste with more salt and pepper. Stir in the sage just before serving in two warm bowls topped with a little more cheese.

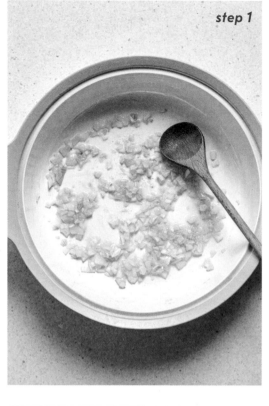

step 1

tip

If you want to go the extra mile, instead of simply chopping the sage and stirring in into the finished risotto you can fry it in a little oil until just crisp for a wonderfully crunchy and aromatic garnish.

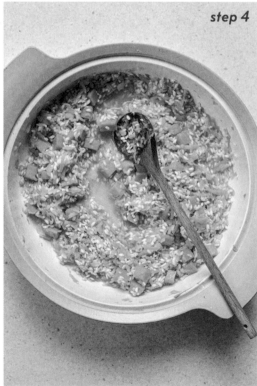

step 4

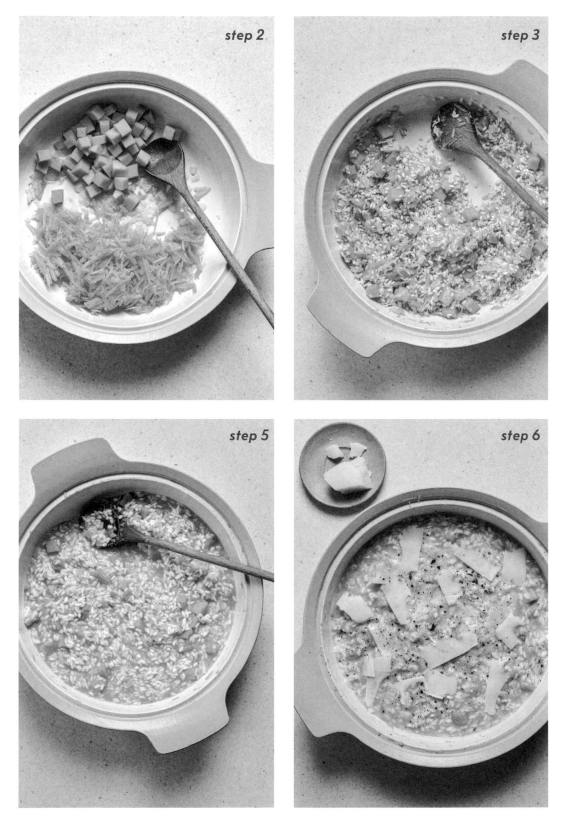

step 2

step 3

step 5

step 6

French Onion Soup with Goats' Cheese Toasts

SERVES 2

Preparation time: 15 minutes
Cooking time: 45 minutes

350g (12oz) onions
large knob of unsalted butter
generous glug of extra virgin
   olive oil
pinch of golden caster sugar
90ml (6 tbsp) white wine
500ml (2 cups) vegetable stock
small handful of fresh thyme, plus
   extra to garnish
glug of brandy or cognac
freshly ground sea salt and black
   pepper

For the goats' cheese
toasts
2 large slices of farmhouse bread
1 large garlic clove
2 small rounds of relatively soft
   goats' cheese

My mum makes the most incredible French onion soup, and I remember when I was little helping her caramelise the onions in her big, heavy blue casserole pot. I never used to cook it for myself because I can't eat the traditional cheese croutons that make it so special, but I can eat goats' cheese, which is how I came to discover this delicious twist on a classic dish.

1. Peel and thinly slice the onions into half-moons using a large, very sharp, very heavy knife, a mandolin or the slicing attachment on your food processor.

2. Heat the butter and olive oil over a medium heat in a large heavy-based saucepan. Once the butter is frothing, add the onions, sugar and a large pinch of sea salt and stir until the onions are coated in the butter and oil. Once you hear the onions sizzling, turn the heat to medium-low, allowing them to caramelise; this should take about half an hour.

3. Turn the heat up to medium-high. Splash in the wine, and, when bubbling, follow with the vegetable stock, thyme and freshly ground black pepper.

4. Bring the pan to the boil, then reduce to simmer for 10 minutes.

5. Meanwhile, make the goats' cheese toasts. Preheat the grill to high. Very lightly toast the bread and halve the garlic clove – don't worry about peeling it! Rub one side of each piece of bread with each garlic half. Slice the cheese, and lay it over the toast so that every inch is covered. Grill for a couple of minutes until the cheese is well melted.

6. Stir in a good glug of brandy and check for seasoning. Serve in hot bowls with a little more fresh thyme and a goats' cheese toast on the side for dunking.

Mexican Baked Eggs

SERVES 2

Preparation time: 5 minutes
Cooking time: 35 minutes

splash of light oil
1 large onion
1 large yellow pepper
1 tbsp chipotle paste
1½ x 400g (14oz) tins chopped
    tomatoes (or use 1 large tin and
    1 small tin)
400g (14oz) tin black beans
4 large eggs
1 large ripe avocado
small handful of fresh coriander
juice of ½ lime
sea salt

Tomato baked eggs seem not to be as popular a brunch dish as they used to be, but I actually think this is a good thing, because it means I can bulk them up a bit, Mexican-style and serve them for dinner, instead of reserving them for weekend breakfasts. Serve with toasted flour tortillas on the side for dipping, and a dollop of soured cream if you find the chipotle-laced tomato sauce a little on the spicy side.

1. Heat the oil in a large, lidded casserole dish over a medium-high heat. Peel and roughly chop the onion then core and deseed the pepper before chopping it into bite-sized pieces. Fry both along with a large pinch of sea salt for 15 minutes or so until everything is soft and slightly charred.

2. Stir the chipotle paste into the pan and cook for a further minute before adding the chopped tomatoes and the drained black beans (don't bother to rinse them).

3. Stir everything well and turn up the heat, bringing the sauce to the boil. The moment it starts to bubble, reduce the heat to medium-low and allow it to simmer for 15 minutes or so, until the sauce has thickened.

4. Check to see if you would like to add any more salt before making four wells in the sauce in to which to crack the eggs. Do so, and put on the lid, leaving the eggs to bake for 4–5 minutes (depending on your pan you may need a little more) until the whites are just set and the yolks are still runny.

5. Meanwhile, peel and cube the avocado and roughly chop the coriander.

6. Scatter the avocado cubes over the pan and squeeze over the lime juice. Sprinkle over the coriander just before serving, still in the casserole dish.

Tomato and Chickpea Alphabet Soup

SERVES 4

Preparation time: 5 minutes
Cooking time: 20 minutes

4 large garlic cloves, thinly sliced
2 tbsp extra virgin olive oil, plus
  extra for drizzling
2 x 400g (14oz) tins chickpeas
2 x 400g (14oz) tins chopped
  tomatoes
800ml (3½ cups) vegetable
  stock
1 Parmesan rind (*make sure you
  use a vegetarian version if this
  matters to you*)
1 bay leaf
large pinch of golden caster
  sugar
100g (3½oz) small pasta shapes
freshly ground sea salt and black
  pepper
fresh rosemary, to serve

Like many of my favourite recipes, this simple take on the Italian classic, pasta e ceci, started off as a commission I carried on tweaking long after publication. *BBC Food* asked me to create a cheap, quick, five-ingredient tomato, chickpea and pasta soup, and I loved it so much I wanted to see what happened if I restored some of the little luxuries that had been stripped out to stick to the five-ingredient brief. The addition of a dried bay leaf adds an extra layer of aromatics, and the little addition of a pinch of sugar rounds the whole thing out nicely. These changes might look like I've simply gilded the lily, but they make a surprisingly big impact.

1. Put the sliced garlic along with the olive oil into the bottom of a large saucepan and set over a medium-high heat. Allow the garlic to infuse into the oil as it heats and the garlic starts to soften. Be sure not to let it brown!

2. Drain the chickpeas and add to the pan with the chopped tomatoes, vegetable stock, Parmesan rind, bay leaf and sugar and stir to combine. Turn up the heat, bringing it to the boil, then reduce the heat to medium-low and season well with salt and pepper.

3. Allow to simmer for 5 minutes before adding the pasta. Simmer for a further 15 minutes, or until the pasta is just tender.

4. Fish out the Parmesan rind and the bay leaf and check the seasoning.

5. Serve in warm bowls topped with a generous drizzle of olive oil and a sprinkling of finely chopped rosemary needles.

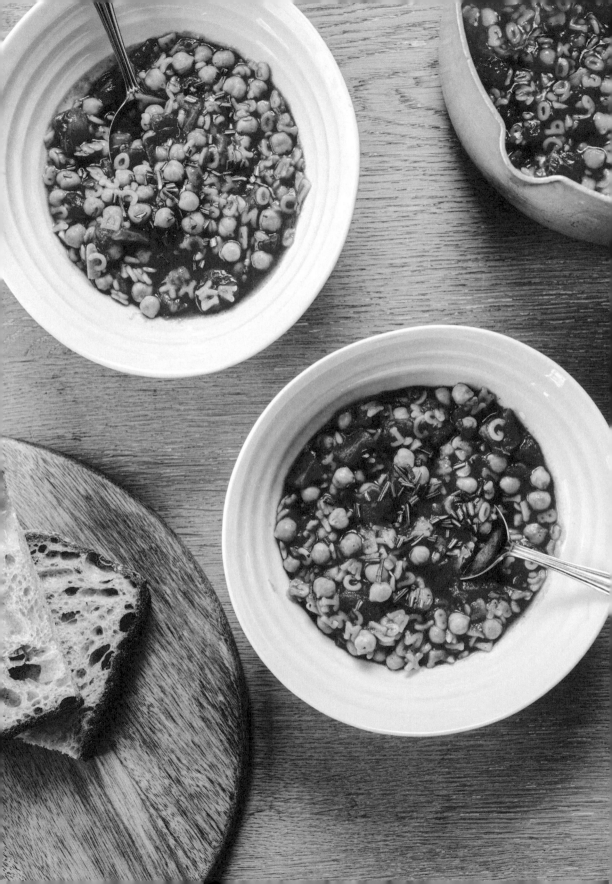

Watermelon, Avocado and Feta Salad with Lime Dressing

SERVES 4

Preparation time: 15 minutes
Cooking time: 5 minutes

2 large handfuls of sunflower
    seeds
4 avocados
1.2kg (2¾lb) watermelon, cubed
2 large handfuls of fresh mint,
    roughly chopped
120g (4oz) feta

For the dressing
zest of 1 lime
juice of 2 limes
2 tbsp extra virgin olive oil
sea salt
golden caster sugar

Sometimes I find watermelons really disappointing; often they've been left too long and their flesh has turned soft rather than crisp, or they simply turn out to be not very sweet. This all changed when I had my first bite of an Italian watermelon. Their flavour is impossibly sweet, and that taste got me excited to get back in the kitchen and create a dish with this wonderful fruit.

This salad is bright and refreshing, perfect for the height of summer. The addition of avocado alongside the crumbled feta makes it filling enough to be enjoyed as a light meal, but it would also make a great side to grilled or barbecued meat or tofu.

1. Toast the sunflower seeds in a small saucepan over a medium heat, tossing occasionally. When the skins start to pop, remove from the heat and set aside.

2. Peel and cube the avocados and add to a large bowl along with the watermelon, mint and toasted sunflower seeds. Crumble over the feta and set aside.

3. To make the dressing, whisk together the lime zest and juice, olive oil, and a couple of good pinches of sea salt and sugar, to taste.

4. Pour the dressing over the salad, and toss together gently to be sure that the feta stays in chunks, and the avocado doesn't get too badly mushed. Set aside for 5 minutes to allow the flavours to meld before serving.

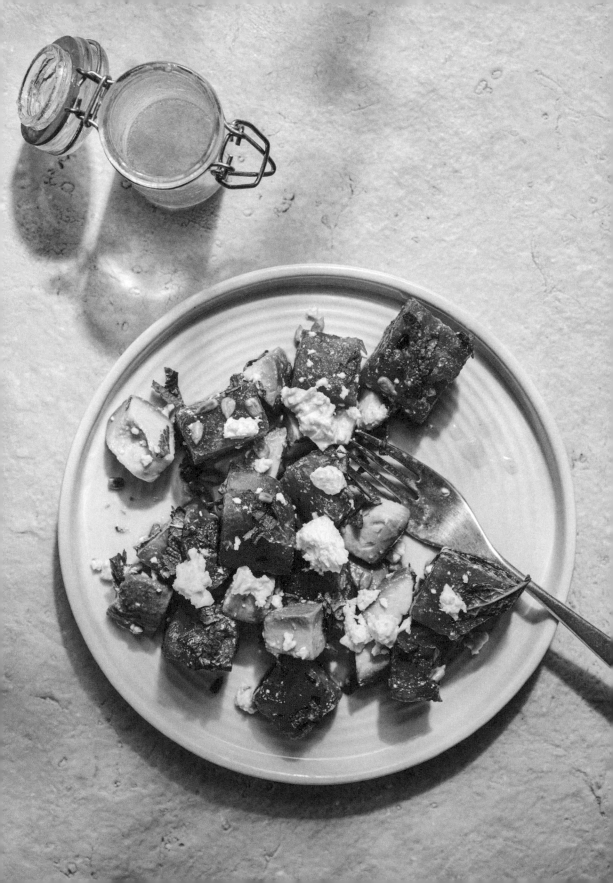

Gigantes Plaki with Feta

SERVES 2–3

Preparation time: 5 minutes
Cooking time: 30 minutes

splash of light oil
1 small onion
1 tsp sea salt
2 large garlic cloves
1 tsp ground cinnamon
1 tbsp tomato purée
400g (14oz) tin chopped
   tomatoes
300g (10oz) tinned or jarred
   butter beans (about 1½ tins,
   drained weight)
1 tsp golden caster sugar
½ tsp dried oregano
½ tsp dried thyme
60ml (4 tbsp) vegetable stock or
   water
60g (2¼oz) feta
small handful of fresh basil, flat
   leaf parsley or fresh oregano
freshly ground black pepper

One of the first things I remember cooking all by myself for my parents while they were working outside in the garden one weekend was gigantes, a big dish of Greek butter beans in a cinnamony tomato sauce, baked to bubbly perfection. Here, I've transformed that baked pan of beans into a simple stovetop supper, piled into warm bowls with crumbled feta and handfuls of basil, and perhaps with some crusty bread to mop up the sauce.

1. Heat the oil in a large saucepan over a medium-high heat. Peel and finely chop the onion, add to the pan with the sea salt and gently fry for 5 minutes or so until soft and just starting to brown. Peel and thinly slice the garlic cloves and add them to the pan, frying for a further minute until they're soft and aromatic, but not yet starting to colour.

2. Stir in the cinnamon and tomato purée and fry for a further minute.

3. Add the chopped tomatoes, butter beans (drained and rinsed), sugar and dried herbs. Use the vegetable stock or water to wash any excess tomato goodness from the tin and add that to the pan too. Season well with black pepper.

4. Turn up the heat to bring the beans to the boil. Reduce the heat to low and allow to simmer, uncovered, for 20 minutes. If the sauce looks a little dry, add a little more stock or water.

5. Check to see if you want to add any more salt or pepper before serving in warm bowls with the crumbled feta and your choice of herb, roughly chopped, sprinkled over the top.

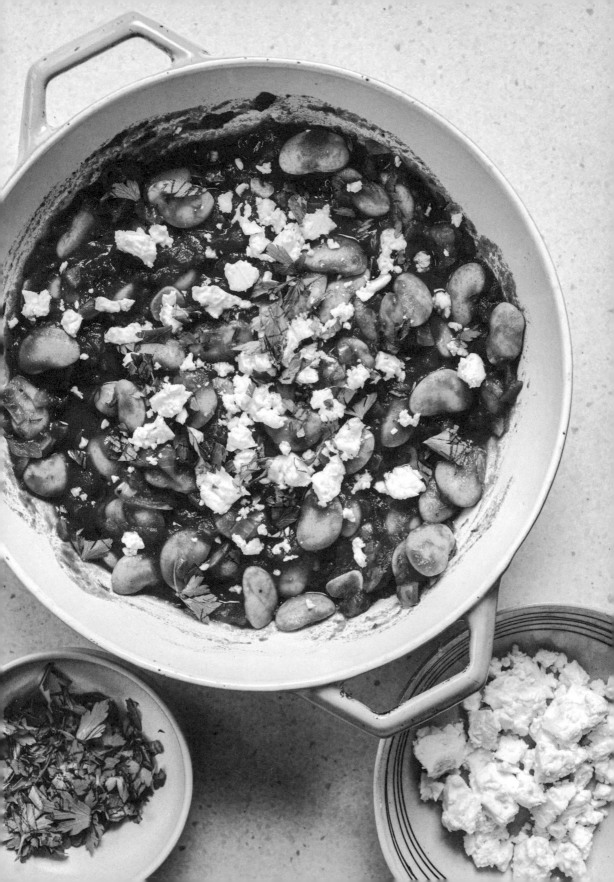

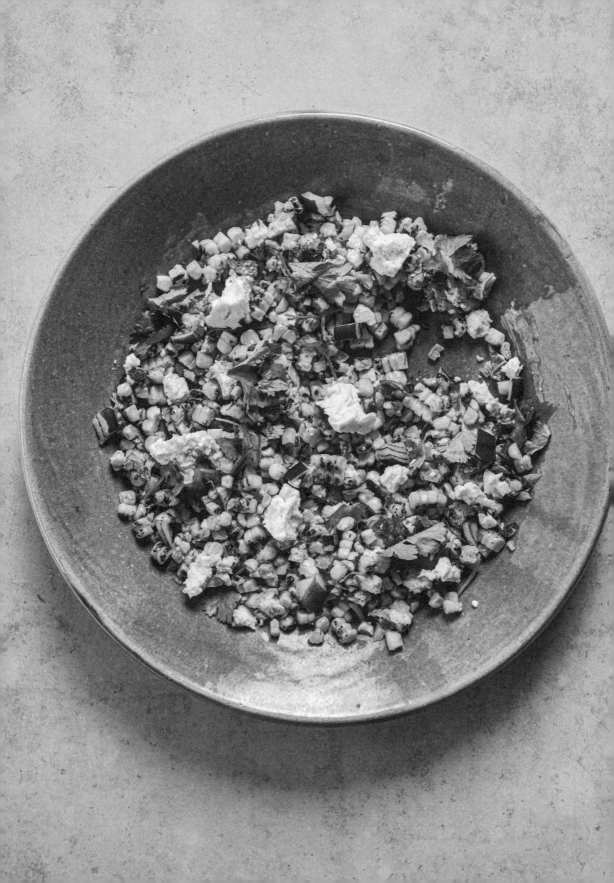

Grilled Mexican Street Corn Salad

SERVES 3–4

Preparation time: 10 minutes
Cooking time: 15 minutes

1 large red onion
4 corn on the cob
very large handful of fresh
   coriander
¼ tsp hot smoked paprika
1–2 tbsp Kewpie mayonnaise
fresh lime juice
120g (4oz) feta
sea salt

My take on the Mexican-street food classic (switching the traditional queso fresco for feta because the former is difficult to find in the UK) is a tasty solo lunch or a side salad for a larger Mexican feast to be enjoyed at the height of summer. More importantly it is part of my ongoing campaign to wean people off tinned sweetcorn and on to the slightly grill-blackened stuff shaved right off the cob.

1. Peel and finely chop the red onion. Leave the pieces to soak in a small bowl of cold water – this will take some of the bite out of the raw onion. Next, heat the barbecue or your griddle pan – you want things smoking hot!

2. Clean the corn cobs if necessary before charring them straight on the griddle for 10–15 minutes, turning regularly, until they're very well charred. Remove from the heat and set aside until they're cool.

3. Meanwhile, drain and pat the onion dry on a piece of kitchen paper and toss in a large bowl with the coriander, roughly chopped.

4. Hold each cob upright with the round flat base resting on the cutting board. Working in a downward sweeping motion, turning the cob a little as you go, use a large sharp knife to shave the corn kernels off the cob.

5. Add the corn to the bowl, and toss together with the paprika and mayonnaise (start with 1 tablespoon and add more if you want things a little creamier) until everything is combined. Season to taste with lime juice and sea salt, and top with the feta, crumbled.

koreatown

It was one single meal that started my love affair with Korean food and flavours.

One afternoon I hopped on an L.A. city bus with a bunch of other study-abroad students with one goal in mind: heading into Koreatown to seek out some traditional Korean barbecue. None of us had eaten Korean food before or even knew much about it, but we found ourselves standing on a corner looking a little lost, and wondering where we could find ourselves something good to eat. I'd just discovered that Yelp gives you restaurant recommendations based on your location, and from there we ended up heading down West 8th Street in the direction of Soot Bull Jeep which remains, to this day, where I experienced one of the very best meals of my life.

Soot Bull Jeep is a traditional Korean barbecue restaurant. It's sparse inside, the only adornments on the tables being the big, open charcoal grills set into the middle of each one. A group of Korean grandmas were gossiping in the corner while they peeled massive bags of fat garlic cloves, and I'm pretty sure we were the only table speaking English. Soot Bull Jeep, it turned out, has something of a cult following among off-duty Korean chefs.

We ended up with three massive bowls of beef, chicken and pork, which came to the table raw and marinated, to cook yourself until tender over the coals. The staff took pity on us and showed us how to do it, though you really are expected to cook everything yourself. They must have known we were out of our depth as we didn't order any rice; we may have been in the middle of health-conscious L.A., but a Korean meal without rice is not a meal, it is simply a snack. The meat was good, but it was the banchan – something we had no idea about at the time – which really had me charmed.

Banchan, little dishes of pickled and prepared vegetables and ferments, are as essential to any Korean meal as the rice I've just mentioned, even in Korean homes. They are usually free in Korean restaurants, though unless you know where to go in London they've become a chargeable item. Sometimes they will just be one or two things found in the fridge given as accompaniments; in some restaurants and at big feasts the entire table can become covered in them. We had pickled daikon, sesame dressed spinach, a spicy spring onion and lettuce salad, a fermented soybean, Doenjang-based dip, crunchy sesame soy beansprouts, and some of those raw garlic cloves the grannies were peeling to char on the grill. At the time we had no idea what any of them were and just used our favourites to build our meal, wiping big lettuce leaves in the soybean paste before piling them up with impossibly flavourful and tender meats, pickles and ferments. All we knew was that everything was absolutely delicious, and we

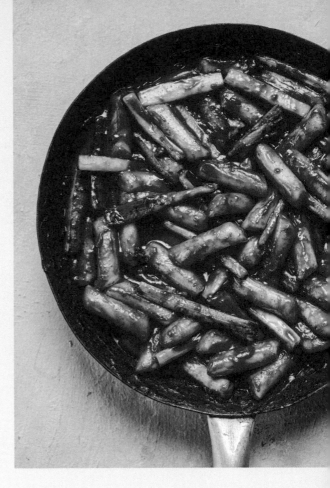

It was the banchan . . . which really had me charmed.

were perfectly content to sit there and stuff ourselves to bursting, even if we had absolutely no idea what we were eating.

Among the banchan there were also a few different dishes of what appeared to me to be a spicy type of tangy, fermented cabbage that I took to immediately. At the time I had no idea what it was. I had discovered kimchee, Korean's national dish, and an ingredient that is now as essential to my fridge as a pat of butter and a jar of French mustard.

I've since learned that some of the very best Korean food in the world can be found in Los Angeles's Koreatown; it is almost entirely cooked by Korean immigrants for fellow Korean immigrants and their families, giving it a solid mark of authenticity, and California simply has much better fresh produce than is commonly available in Korea. No wonder I fell so deeply in love.

When I returned to England Korean cooking was still pretty rare, but traditional Korean ingredients such as ready-made kimchee, gochujang (a type of fermented, soy-based chilli paste) and toasted sesame oil were much easier to find in Asian supermarkets, so I started breaking out on my own, first perfecting a couple of traditional Korean dishes, and then later starting to add Korean flavours to other things. If you want a taste of almost-traditional Korean cooking try my **Kimchee Fried Rice** over the page, my **Spicy Korean Rice Cakes** (page 146) and my **Korean Sashimi Salad** (page 156). For a little taste of Korean fusion, try my **Pea and Courgette Burgers with Kimchee** (page 78) and my **Korean Salmon with Sesame Veggies** (page 215), or simply pile some kimchee on to your next piece of avocado toast.

Kimchee Fried Rice

SERVES 2

Preparation time: 5 minutes
Cooking time: 30 minutes

2 large eggs
4 tsp light oil
160g (1 cup) kimchee
1 tbsp gochujang
2 tsp dark soy sauce
2 x 250g (9oz) pouches brown
  rice
4 large spring onions
1 tsp toasted sesame oil

Kimchee Fried Rice is my all-time favourite comfort food. If you've never had kimchee or made Korean food before, it is the perfect dish to start off with; I've successfully fed this to kimchee haters as the tangy flavour of the fermented cabbage is somewhat softened as you slightly caramelise. Sometimes I like to keep things plain, but at others I top my bowl with any combination of Kewpie mayonnaise, sriracha, furikake, shreds of nori seaweed and even another egg, fried in toasted sesame oil to give the white deliciously crisp edges.

1. Lightly beat the eggs. Heat half the oil in a large non-stick frying pan or a wok over a medium heat. 500g (1lb 2oz) is a lot of cooked rice, so make sure your pan is big enough to accommodate it all before you start!

2. Then add the eggs and scramble until just cooked and broken up into small pieces before transferring to a bowl.

3. Roughly chop the kimchee. Heat the rest of the oil in the pan until shimmering, and gently fry the kimchee and any excess juices for a few minutes until the cabbage is fragrant, slightly translucent and is just starting to caramelise.

4. Stir the gochujang and soy sauce into the fried kimchee until combined before stirring in the rice. If you are using pre-cooked pouches of rice, I find the easiest way to separate the grains is to gently massage the pouches before you open them.

5. Make sure the rice is well coated in the kimchee mixture, then return the egg to the pan. Thinly slice the spring onions and add, cooking everything until the rice and the egg pieces are heated through.

6. Remove the pan from the heat and stir through the toasted sesame oil before serving.

tip

I'm using pouch rice here for ease, but you can also use cooked brown basmati rice, leftover Asian-style rice or even riced cauliflower.

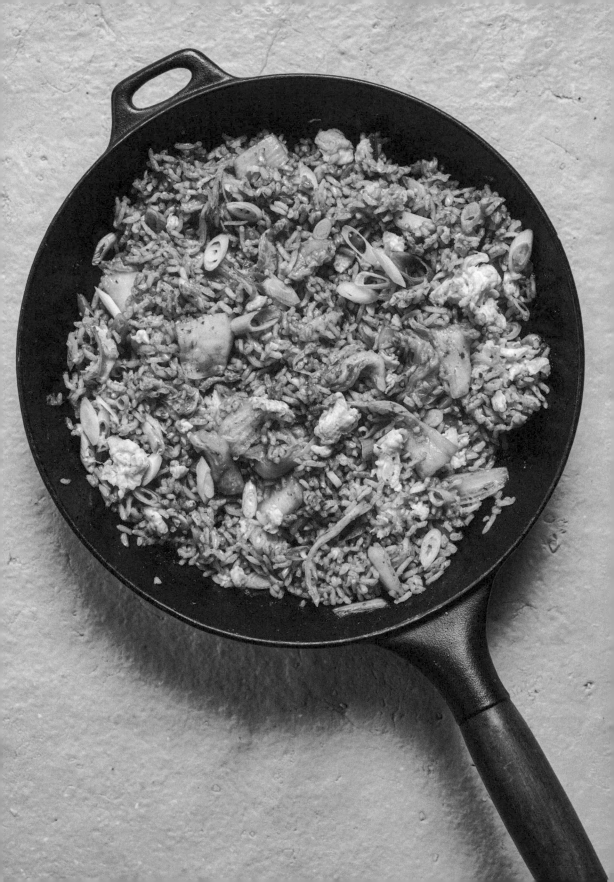

Pea and Courgette Burgers with Kimchee

SERVES 3-4

Preparation time: 10 minutes
Cooking time: 15 minutes

1 courgette
½ tsp sea salt
1 large egg
3 tbsp plain flour
½ tsp baking powder
freshly ground black pepper
small handful of frozen petit pois,
    defrosted
light oil, for frying

To serve
3–4 burger buns
Kewpie mayonnaise
kimchee

My friend Natasha lives in Paris, where she writes fantastic, bestselling young adult fantasy fiction. Just before she made the big move across the Channel a couple of us got together for leaving drinks at the bar of the National Theatre on London's South Bank. We ate from the food trucks parked outside, and I had an amazing veggie burger with a difference, which has stuck with me ever since. It was a plump, juicy courgette and pea fritter stuffed into a bun along with a generous amount of kimchee and special sauce. Naturally I quickly recreated it at home, again loading up on the kimchee and substituting in my beloved Japanese Kewpie mayo for the burger sauce.

1. On the largest hole of your box grater, grate the courgette into a small bowl. Toss with the sea salt and set aside.

2. To make the batter, whisk together the egg, flour, baking powder and a generous amount of freshly ground black pepper in a small bowl until you've made a smooth paste. Then add the petit pois and mix in well.

3. Heat a large frying pan over a medium-high heat with enough oil to just cover the bottom. Spoon the courgette mixture into the pan to make 3–4 fritters, about the size of your burger buns, and gently fry until they're cooked through and golden on each side, working in batches if necessary. Set the cooked fritters aside on a plate lined with kitchen paper to soak up any excess oil.

4. Split the burger buns and spread each generously with Kewpie mayo. Stuff each with a fritter and a couple of pieces of kimchee. Serve immediately.

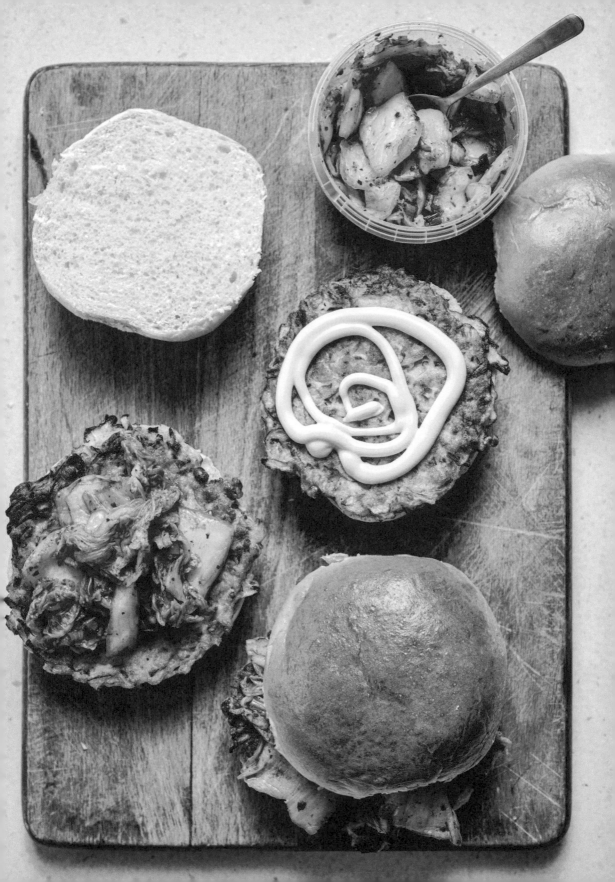

Tofu Bánh Mì Sandwich

SERVES 2–3

Preparation time: 15 minutes,
plus marinating time
Cooking time: 5 minutes

**For the quick
Vietnamese pickles**
1 small carrot
3–4 radishes
2 tbsp rice wine vinegar
¼ tsp sea salt
¼ tsp golden caster sugar

For the Vietnamese tofu
1 large garlic clove
1 tbsp soy sauce
1 tbsp lime juice
1 tsp grated ginger
1 tsp lemongrass paste
1 tsp maple syrup
280g (9½oz) extra-firm tofu

**For the Bánh Mì
sandwiches**
2–3 small baguettes
Kewpie mayonnaise
sriracha hot sauce
large handful of fresh coriander
  leaves

This is one of the best sandwiches I've ever made. It is filling enough to enjoy for dinner and, made with firm tofu instead of the traditional pork, totally veggie. Bánh Mì is a traditionally Vietnamese treat; marinated pork stuffed into a French-style baguette spread with pâté and mayonnaise, loaded up with fresh herbs and pickles. I've tried a couple from street food vendors but none of them have lived up to the mouth-watering description in Uyen Luu's wonderful book *My Vietnamese Kitchen*. This version is more than yummy enough for me to enjoy while I chase that meaty utopia.

1. First, make your pickles. Peel and thinly slice the carrot into matchsticks and top, tail and thinly slice the radishes. Toss together in a small bowl with the rice wine vinegar, sea salt and sugar and set aside for an hour to marinate.

2. To marinate the tofu, peel and crush the garlic and whisk together with the soy sauce, lime juice, ginger, lemongrass paste and maple syrup in a shallow dish. Slice the tofu into thick slices (perfect for stuffing into a split baguette) and submerge in the marinade. Set aside until it is time to assemble the sandwiches.

3. Heat a large, non-stick frying pan or griddle pan over a medium-high heat. Meanwhile, split the baguettes down the middle and spread them generously with Kewpie mayonnaise.

4. Griddle the tofu slices until each side is slightly crisp and caramelised. Stuff the slices into the baguettes, along with a handful of pickles, drained from their pickling liquid and patted dry on a piece of kitchen paper, a good squirt of sriracha and some coriander leaves. Eat immediately.

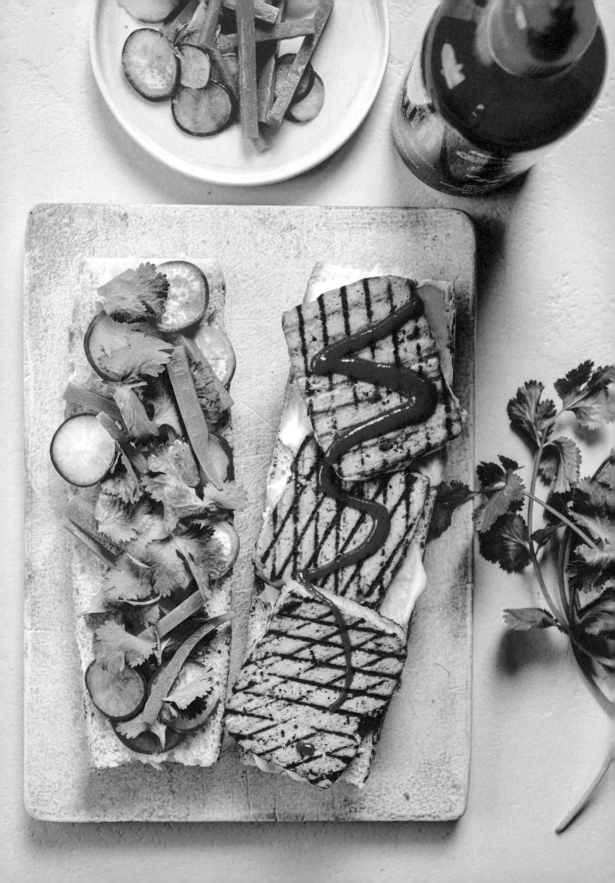

Coconut Curry Zoodles with Asian Greens and Silken Tofu

SERVES 2

Preparation time: 10 minutes
Cooking time: 10 minutes

2 garlic cloves
2 tsp grated ginger
4 spring onions
2 tbsp light oil
3 tbsp Southeast Asian curry
   paste
300ml (1¼ cups) light coconut
   milk
500ml (2 cups) vegetable stock
1 tsp runny honey
1 tsp fish sauce (*or soy sauce for a
   vegetarian option*)
2 small courgettes
large handful of sugar snap peas
2 baby pak choi
1 red chilli
160g (5¼oz) silken tofu
lime wedges, for serving

The key to creating the perfect bowl of Southeast Asian noodles or courgette noodles is to fry off a few aromatics before adding curry paste to the pan to make sure you get a complex, layered broth, regardless of the paste you're using. I love the Peranakan Turmeric & Lemongrass Spice Paste from Rempapa Spice Co.

1. Peel and crush the garlic, peel and grate the ginger and thinly slice the spring onions.

2. Heat the oil in a large saucepan over a medium-high heat. Once the oil is shimmering, add the garlic, ginger and spring onions and fry for about a minute until they're just starting to colour. Add the curry paste and cook for another couple of minutes until the paste has softened slightly and everything is smelling lovely and aromatic.

3. Stir in the coconut milk, followed by the vegetable stock, honey and fish or soy sauce. Reduce the broth to a low simmer while you prepare the rest of the ingredients.

4. Using a spiraliser, break the courgette down into noodles (I find a small hand-held one the easiest to use – mine looks a bit like a pencil sharpener – but you can also create courgette noodles by running the length of the courgette down the largest hold of a box grater repeatedly in a single motion.) Roughly chop the rest of the veggies, adding them all to the simmering liquid as and when they're ready.

5. Thinly slice the chilli and cut the tofu into small cubes before dividing the soup between two large, warm bowls and adding them both over the top. Serve with a couple of lime wedges for spritzing.

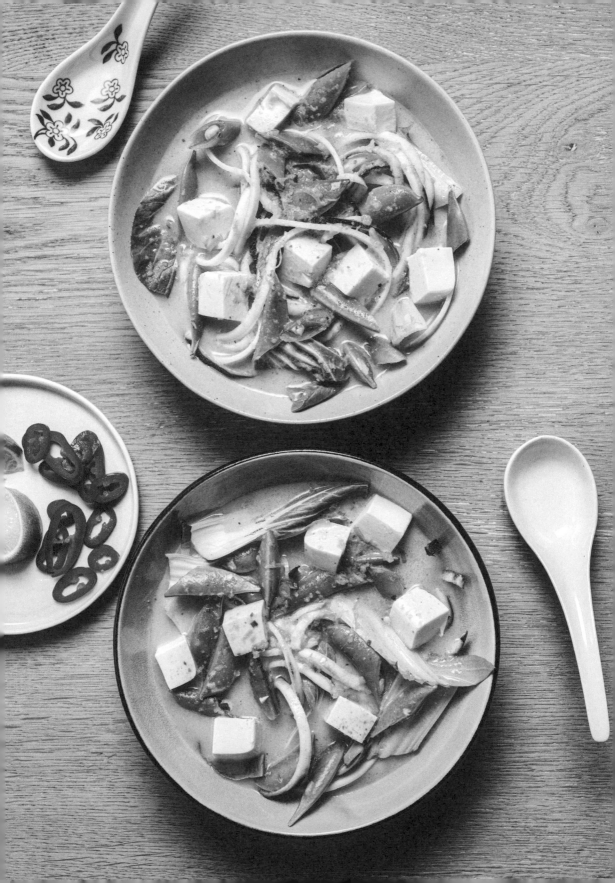

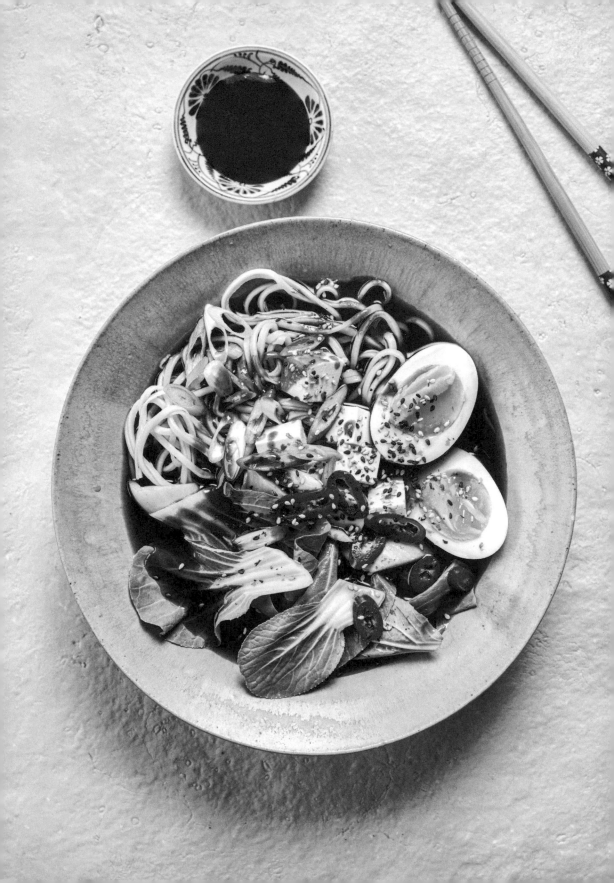

Slow Cooker Ramen

SERVES 2

Preparation time: 10 minutes
Cooking time: 4–8 hours

For the broth
750ml (3 cups) fresh vegetable
    stock
4cm (1½in) fresh ginger
2 large garlic cloves
1½ tbsp dark soy sauce
1 tbsp rice wine vinegar
1 tsp red miso paste

For the ramen
2 baby pak choi
2 nests of ramen noodles
2 large eggs (*optional*)
½ red chilli
2 large spring onions
50g (2oz) cubed silken tofu
furikake, to sprinkle
your favourite hot sauce, to serve
    (*I often use the leftover sauce
    from the **Korean Sashimi
    Salad** on page 156*)

tip

*Use any leftover tofu to make
the **Tex-Mex Tofu Scramble** on
page 124.*

It turns out that the secret to getting a deep and flavourful broth to use as the base for a steaming bowl of homemade ramen is to make it in the slow cooker. You can set the soup to infuse while you're at work, just adding the noodles and veggies – and boiling an egg if you want – when you get home. Ramen is a great weeknight way to clear the fridge, and can be made vegan by omitting the soft-boiled egg, or meaty by adding some shredded leftover roast duck, chicken, pork or beef.

1. To make the broth, combine the vegetable stock, ginger (sliced into coins), garlic cloves (lightly smashed using the end of a rolling pin – no need to peel them), soy sauce, rice wine vinegar and miso paste in your slow cooker and cook on high for 4 hours, or on low for 8 hours. Alternatively, bring all the ingredients to the boil in a large, lidded saucepan before reducing to a very low simmer and leaving to infuse, covered, for an hour.

2. When you are ready to eat, prepare the ramen. Thickly slice the pak choi and add it to the slow cooker or saucepan along with the noodles. Cook on low for 15 minutes, or until the noodles are tender.

3. Meanwhile, boil the eggs, if using, for 6 minutes before plunging them in cold water to stop them cooking. Carefully peel and halve once they are cool enough to handle. Thinly slice the chilli and spring onions.

4. Divide the noodles, pak choi and broth between two bowls. Top with the halved eggs, red chilli and spring onion slices, the tofu cubes and a sprinkling of furikake. Bring the hot sauce to the table so that people can drizzle it over themselves.

Cheat's Dhal Makhani

SERVES 2
**(OR 4–6 AS PART OF
AN INDIAN MEAL)**

Preparation time: 5 minutes
Cooking time: 20 minutes

2 small onions
2 large garlic clove
30g (1oz) fresh ginger
2 tbsp light oil
1 tbsp garam masala
1 tsp ground turmeric
1 tsp sweet smoked paprika
½ tsp chilli powder
120ml (½ cup) passata
1 tsp salt
2 x 400ml (14oz) tins beluga
   lentils
200ml (¾ cup) single cream
30g (2 tbsp) unsalted butter
chopped fresh coriander, to
   garnish (*optional*)

I'm a creature of habit so whenever we get a curry I always order dhal makhani to go along with our shared sides for a lamb biriyani – a peshwari naan and sometimes a spoonful of Bombay potatoes; it is one of my ultimate comfort foods. If I want to make it myself, I always turn to this cheat's dhal which is much better suited to weeknights than some traditional recipes. Instead of simmering the lentils for hours I get them out of a tin, and I've switched the whole spices for ground, before finishing the whole thing off with the traditional slug of cream and slick of butter.

1. Peel and roughly chop the onions, garlic and ginger before blitzing in a mini chopper. If you don't have one, chop everything as finely as you can manage!

2. Heat the oil in a large, heavy-bottomed saucepan or casserole over a medium heat. Add the blitzed paste and gently fry for 5–6 minutes until it has turned translucent and just starting to brown.

3. Stir in the spices and cook for a further minute, making sure they don't burn – you'll know if this is the case because they'll darken and stick to the pot; if this happens all you can do is throw the whole lot out and start again as you'll taste it in the final dhal!

4. Add the passata, 200ml water, salt and drained lentils – you don't need to worry about rinsing them.

5. Allow the mixture to simmer for 5 minutes before stirring in most of the cream (save a spoonful for serving), followed by the butter. Give it a taste to see if you want to add any more salt and let it simmer for another 5 minutes, or until the lentils have reached your preferred consistency.

6. Serve in a bowl with warm naan on the side for dunking, a swirl of cream and a sprinkle of coriander.

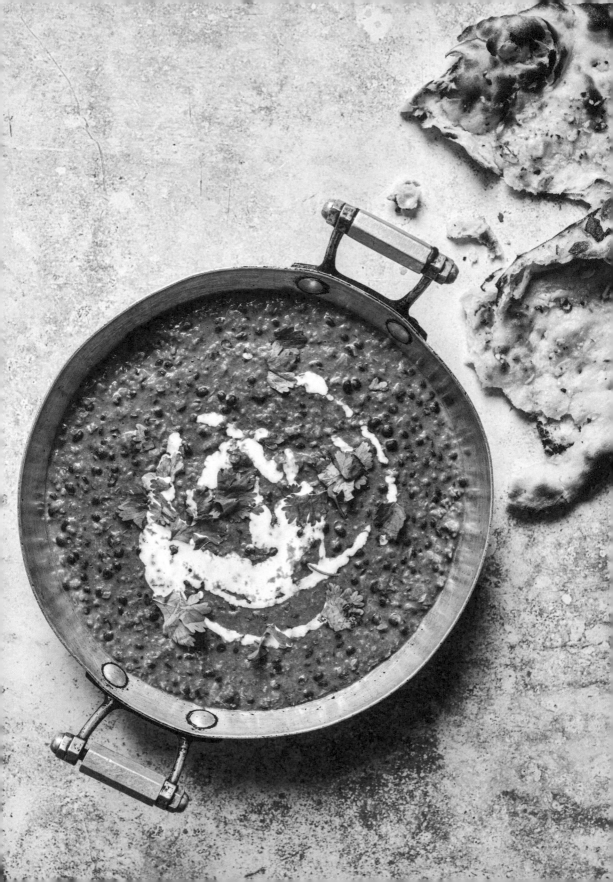

Cheat's Chaat Salad

SERVES 2–4

Preparation time: 10 minutes
Cooking time: 10–15 minutes

200g (7oz) potatoes
1 large spring onion
100g (½ cup) cherry tomatoes
400g (14oz) tin chickpeas
large handful of pomegranate
    seeds
small handful of fresh coriander
½ tsp garam masala
½ tsp sea salt
¼ tsp chilli powder
juice of roughly ¼ lemon, to taste
3 tbsp yogurt
3 tsp tamarind paste
mango chutney, to serve

Whether I'm eating out or at home I always like something fresh and bright to cut through the richer curries on my plate. Enter this Cheat's Chaat Salad, a totally inauthentic, but still very delicious mash up of genuinely authentic chaat recipes I've found online. I love to serve it both as part of an Indian feast or as a big lunchtime treat for two.

1. Peel and chop the potatoes into small cubes. Transfer to a small saucepan of cold, salted water and set over a high heat. Bring to the boil and cook the potatoes for 10–15 minutes until they're only just tender – don't let them fall apart! Drain, and set aside.

2. Finely chop the spring onion and cherry tomatoes. Combine with the rinsed and drained chickpeas, pomegranate seeds (setting a few aside for the garnish) and most of the coriander, roughly chopped. Add the garam masala, salt, chilli powder and a generous squeeze of fresh lemon juice and fold together, making sure everything is well coated.

3. Fold in the potatoes, very gently, making sure they get well coated in the spice mixture but don't fall apart. Check the seasoning to see if you want to add any more salt or lemon juice, then transfer to a serving dish.

4. Mix together the yogurt and tamarind paste and drizzle over the chaat, along with some mango chutney. Finish the dish with the remaining pomegranate seeds and coriander before serving at room temperature.

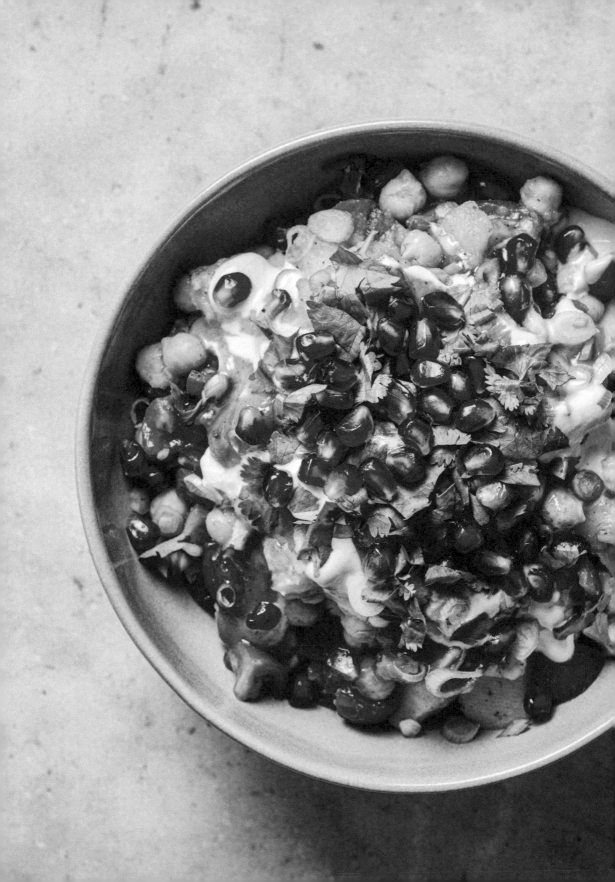

Dhal Baked Eggs
with Chickpeas

SERVES 2

Preparation time: 5 minutes
Cooking time: 55 minutes

1 small white onion
1 large garlic clove
splash of light oil
½ tsp sea salt
½ tsp dried chilli flakes, plus
  extra for sprinkling
½ tsp ground cumin
¼ tsp ground turmeric
150g (¾ cup) red split lentils
100ml (6 tbsp) passata
600ml (2½ cup) vegetable stock
400g (14oz) tin chickpeas
4 large eggs
freshly ground black pepper
  (*optional*)

This is one of the most soothing South Indian-inspired
suppers I can think of. Red split lentils were one of the
first 'new' ingredients I started cooking with as a student.
Here they're gently simmered in gentle spices and strained
tomatoes before being bulked out with tender chickpeas to
form a delicious base for baked eggs. I serve this by itself in
a warm bowl I can get my hands around, and some warm
naan for dipping and scooping never goes amiss here.

1. Peel and finely chop the onion and the garlic clove. Heat the
   oil in a casserole dish or large, lidded, non-stick frying pan
   over a medium-high heat. Add the onions and salt and fry for
   about 5 minutes until they're softened and only just starting to
   brown.

2. Add the garlic and fry for a further minute until fragrant, then
   add the spices, frying for another minute more.

3. Rinse the lentils in a large sieve under the cold tap until the
   water runs clear. Drain and add them to the pan, stirring for a
   minute or so until they've heated through.

4. Stir in the passata, then the vegetable stock. Turn up the heat
   and bring the pan to the boil. Once the lentils are bubbling
   away, reduce the heat to low and allow them to simmer
   gently, uncovered, for 35–40 minutes, stirring occasionally,
   until almost all the liquid is absorbed and the lentils are
   tender. Check the seasoning to see if you want to add a little
   more salt.

5. Stir in the chickpeas and, with a wooden spoon, make four
   wells in the lentil mixture. Crack the eggs into the wells then
   put on the lid and keeping the heat low, bake the eggs for
   4–5 minutes until the whites are set and the yolks are still
   runny. Don't worry if they take any longer; a large egg takes 5

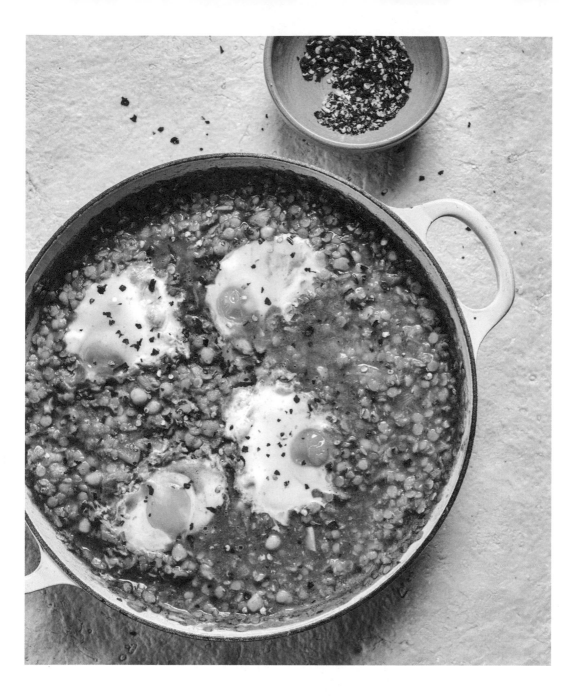

minutes to boil in water so you won't overcook the yolk. Check the eggs after 4 minutes (on some hobs I've seen the eggs in this recipe take up to 10 minutes, so just keep an eye on them).

6. Bring the pan to the table, finished with a simple sprinkling of dried chilli flakes and perhaps a few grinds of black pepper.

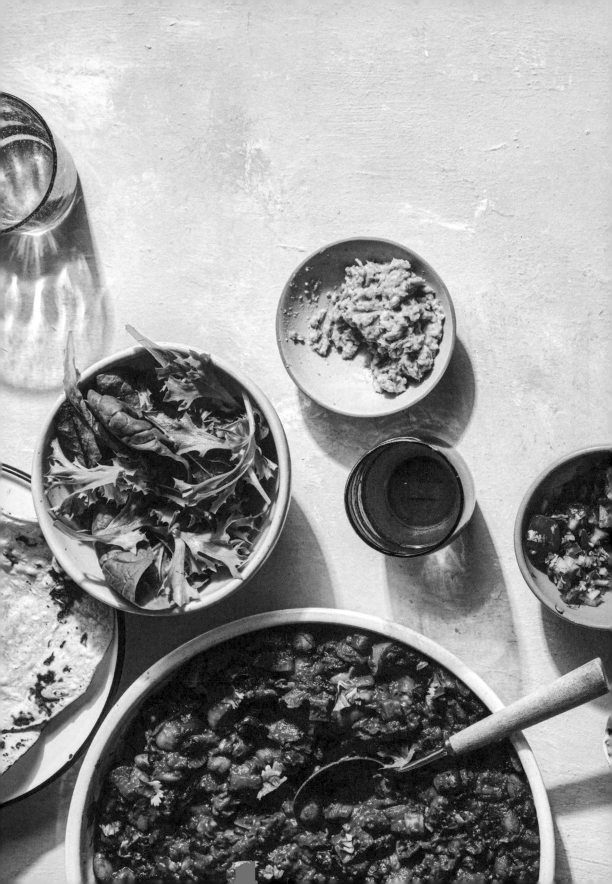

VEGAN

Every summer, I cook a big dinner for our little 'group' at my parents' house near where we all went to school. This year, because I spent the summer writing the book, I'm planning a cosy Bonfire Night supper instead. I'm thinking bangers-in-buns covered in caramelised onions, homemade marshmallows to toast over the bonfire and a big pot of chilli at the centre, obviously accompanied by all the toppings... In recent years, the invitation has extended to an assorted group of girlfriends, boyfriends and parents, and then, a few years ago, one of my closest friends told me that his boyfriend was a vegan, and panic set in. The idea that I'd either have to serve everyone vegan food (I could think of at least four specific people around that table who simply would not stand for the obvious lack of meat) or have the added stress of cooking an entirely separate meal for them just seemed too much.

The truth is, while vegan recipes can be intimidating, they can also be exciting. Which is why it came as something of a surprise to me that this chapter has been the one I've most enjoyed writing. Almost all of my most loved recipes in this book have their home here – including my **Tomato and Root Veggie Casserole with Herby Dumplings** over the page, my **Spicy, Herby Two Pouch Mujadara** (page 108) and my **Vegan Watermelon Poke Bowl** (page 115). You can find what I think is also the most important recipe in this book here: **Slow Cooker Vegetable Stock** (page 99), which forms the backbone of a good many other of the recipes in this book. Yes, I do keep vegetable stock cubes on hand at home too, but nothing beats the homemade stuff.

Just a note of caution here, however. All of the recipes in this chapter are both completely plant-based and very, very tasty, but if you follow an exclusively vegan diet (and you probably know this already) they're coming from a meat eater so they won't necessarily cover all the nutritional bases you need if you have gone strictly vegan, so do make sure they help, rather than hinder you in getting all the nutrients you need each day to enjoy a healthy, balanced diet.

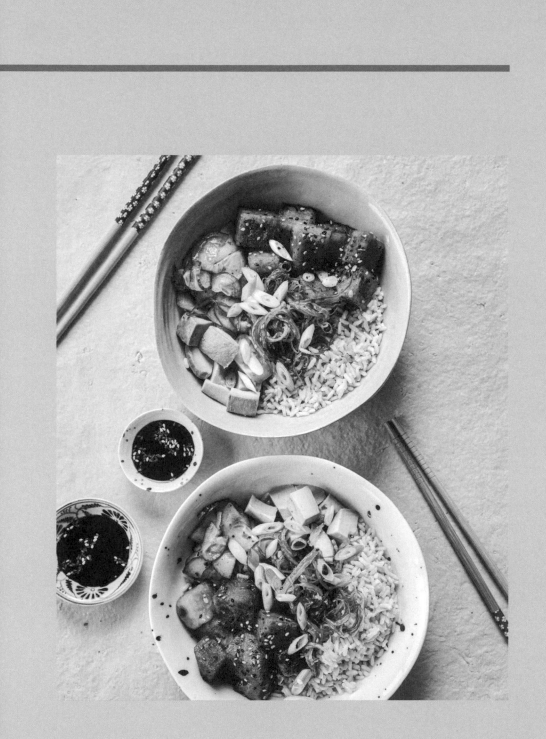

Tomato and Root Veggie Casserole with Herby Dumplings

SERVES 2

Preparation time: 15 minutes
Cooking time: 1 hour 5 minutes

For the root vegetable casserole
1 large leek
1 large parsnip
1 large carrot
1 small swede (about 200g/7oz)
1 sweet potato
1 large garlic clove
1 tbsp light oil
1 tsp dried thyme
400g (14oz) tin chopped
   tomatoes
200ml (¾ cup) vegetable stock
1 tsp vegan-friendly
   Worcestershire sauce
freshly ground sea salt and black
   pepper

For the herby dumplings
65g (½ cup) plain flour
½ tbsp chopped fresh thyme
½ tbsp chopped fresh parsley
30g (¼ cup) vegetable suet
large pinch sea salt
4 tbsp water

This rich, satisfying casserole topped with herby dumplings is what I made one day when I was craving that light, fluffy and uniquely satisfying mouthful you can only really get from a good English dumpling, but I couldn't find any cubed steak to make my usual casserole. It turns out that I actually prefer this accidentally vegan version.

To make this dish truly plant-based you need to use vegetable suet and a vegan-friendly brand of Worcestershire sauce, but if, like me, you're simply seeking to cut down on your meat consumption, you can use beef suet and regular sauce; in terms of taste, you honestly can't tell the difference!

1. Preheat the oven to 200°C/400°F/Gas 6.

2. Top and tail the leek and rinse the top as best you can between the leaves. Cut into roughly 2cm (¾in) lengths. Peel and roughly chop the parsnip, the carrot, swede and the sweet potato. Peel and thinly slice the garlic.

3. Heat the oil over a medium heat in a small, lidded, heavy-based casserole dish or saucepan with an ovenproof handle. Add the leek and cook for about 5 minutes until it has started to soften and take on a good amount of colour around the edges.

4. Add the rest of the root veggies and the sliced garlic to the pot. Cook for a further 10 minutes, turning the heat down to medium-low, allowing the vegetables to soften.

5. Stir in the dried thyme and chopped tomatoes, then use the vegetable stock to rinse the remaining tomato juices out of the tins so that you don't miss out on any of their flavour. Add to the pan with the Worcestershire sauce and a generous amount of salt and pepper.

Continued overleaf . . .

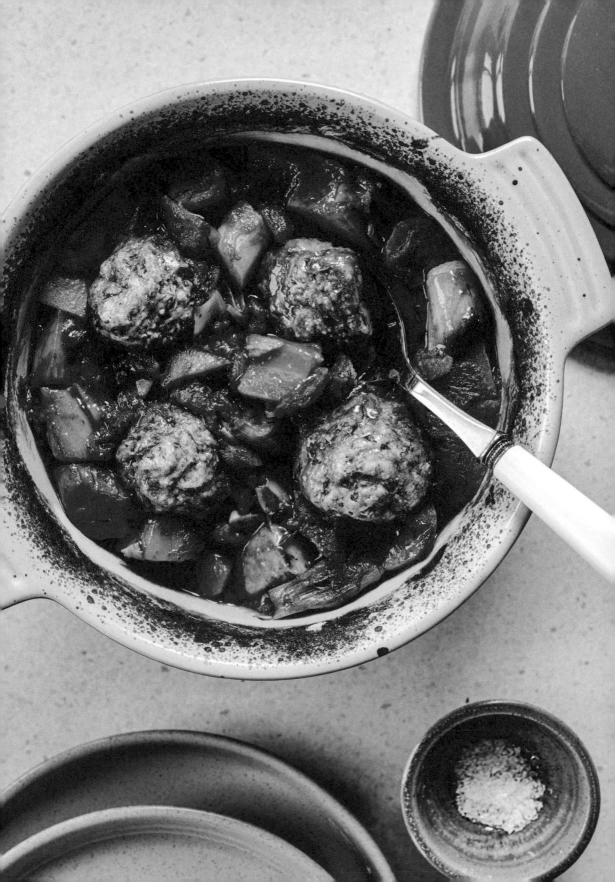

6. Turn the heat up to high and bring the casserole to the boil. Put on the lid and transfer the casserole to the oven to cook for 40 minutes.

7. To make the dumplings, simply combine all of the dry ingredients in a bowl, then mix in the water with a fork until you've created a craggy dough.

8. After 40 minutes, remove the casserole from the oven and set the lid aside. Taste to see if it needs any more salt or pepper. If it looks like there is not enough liquid, feel free to stir in a little water until your casserole has reached your preferred consistency.

9. Using a sharp knife, divide the dumpling dough into four. Flour your hands and shape the dough into rough balls, dropping each into the casserole as you go.

10. Return the casserole to the oven for 20 minutes, uncovered, until the dumplings have puffed up and are slightly golden.

11. Divide between warm bowls and serve immediately.

tip

If you only have just thyme or parsley for the dumplings, don't go out and buy the herb you're missing – just double the quantity of the herb you do have!

Slow Cooker Vegetable Stock

MAKES ABOUT 1 LITRE (4 CUPS)

Preparation time: 5 minutes
Cooking time: 9 hours, or overnight

splash of light oil
1 onion
2 celery sticks
1 leek
2 carrots
1 dried bay leaf
10 black peppercorns

I've been making homemade stock for years. I was originally taught how to put the bones from a roast chicken or our Christmas turkey into a massive, heavy cast-iron casserole dish with some aromatics before covering the whole lot with cold water and leaving it overnight in the warming oven of the Aga. I love this way of turning something that would otherwise be wasted into something useful and versatile so now I use my slow cooker to make stock all the time. When I'm after some homemade stock to use in veggie and vegan dishes, I make this vegetable-based version. These measurements are just a guide; use this recipe to use up odds, ends and peelings of whatever veggies you have, except for parsnips as they will obliterate the nice, clear flavour!

1. Remove the metal insert from your slow cooker and add a splash of oil, setting it over a medium-high heat.

2. Peel and roughly chop the onion, along with the celery, leek and carrots. Gently fry the vegetables until they're just starting to soften around the edges – this should take about 15 minutes.

3. Return the insert to your slow cooker and add the aromatics. Top the whole thing with 1 litre of cold water and set to low for 9 hours, or simply leave it on overnight.

4. Strain away the vegetables and allow the stock to cool completely before freezing. If you use the ice-cube technique, silicone ice-cube trays do the job the best, and you can work in batches storing the frozen cubes in a freezer bag afterwards; if you freeze in tubs, remember to measure out the stock and write the volumes on them so you know which to defrost for which soup recipe! Alternatively, use the stock straight away.

Velvet Vegan Leek and Potato Soup

SERVES 4

Preparation time: 5 minutes
Cooking time: 30 minutes

3 leeks (about 380g/13oz)
2 tbsp extra virgin olive oil, plus
   extra for drizzling
380g (13oz) potatoes
small handful of dill
1 litre (4 cups) vegetable stock
freshly ground sea salt and black
   pepper

This soup exists because I had been researching vegan alternatives to finishing smooth soups with a slick of butter for extra creaminess. One day, inside my charity shop copy of Julia Child's *Mastering the Art of French Cooking*, I found some recipe notes in my own handwriting that I can't remember making for a classic leek and potato soup, which seemed like a good place to start. This soup is finished with a generous glug of extra virgin olive oil to give it that velvety finish, plus a handful of fresh chopped dill.

1. Trim the leeks, and rinse them under the cold tap, gently spreading the leaves at the dark green tops to make sure you wash out any traces of grit from between the leaves. Chop the leeks into roughly 3–4 cm (1½in) rounds.

2 Heat half the olive oil in a large saucepan set over a medium heat. Add the leeks and a large pinch of sea salt and cook for about 10 minutes until the leeks have started to soften and slightly caramelise around the edges.

3. Meanwhile, peel the potatoes and chop them into rough, bite-sized cubes. Finely chop the dill, reserving a few fronds to garnish.

4. Stir the potatoes into the leeks and pour over the stock. Turn up the heat and bring the pan to the boil. Reduce the heat again to low and allow the soup to simmer for 20 minutes, or until the potatoes are tender and falling apart.

5. Remove the soup from the heat and use a hand-held blender to blitz until velvety smooth. Season to taste with salt and pepper and blend in the remaining 1 tablespoon of olive oil.

6. Stir in the dill and serve straight away. Add an extra couple of dill fronds and a swirl of olive oil on top of each bowl.

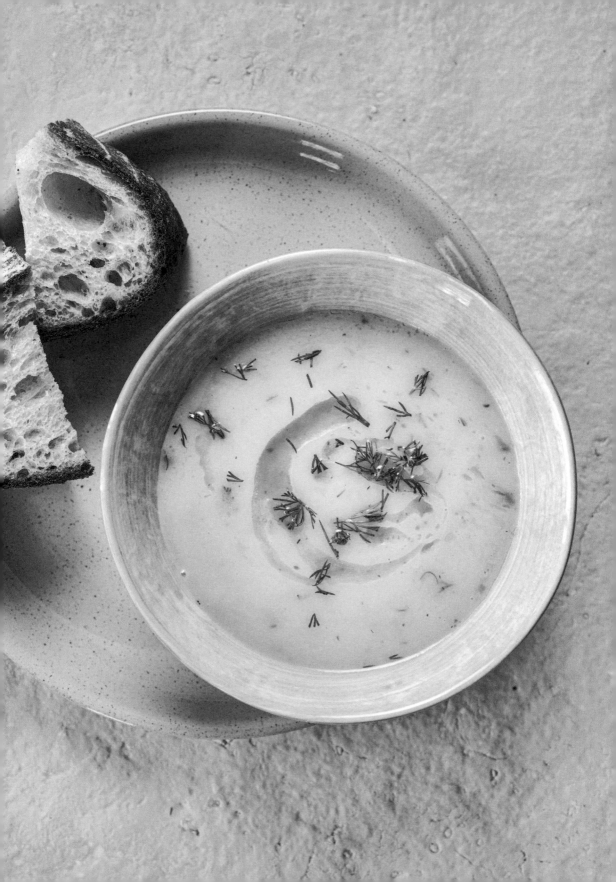

Roasted Autumn Veg with Maple Mustard Dressing

SERVES 1–2

Preparation time: 10 minutes
Cooking time: 30 minutes

200g (7oz) butternut squash
1 small sweet potato
1 large carrot
1 red onion
1 large eating apple
1 tbsp light or garlic-infused oil
freshly ground sea salt and black
  pepper

For the dressing
2½ tsp apple cider vinegar
1½ tsp wholegrain mustard
1½ tsp maple syrup
1½ tsp extra virgin olive oil
small handful of fresh flat leaf
  parsley

This is one of those warm salads that would be great as a side dish to a Sunday roast but is equally delicious by itself for a meat-free midweek meal. I think the combination of butternut squash, sweet potato and roasted apple pieces, still in their skins, looks like autumn leaves and reminds me of those photos you see of New England in the fall, which is what inspired the maple, mustard and apple cider vinegar dressing I've tossed this riot of orange in.

1. Preheat the oven to 200°C/400°F/Gas 6.

2. Peel the butternut squash, sweet potato, carrot and red onion and core the apple. Cut everything except the carrots into bite-sized pieces: cut the carrots into rings that are just over 1cm on the diagonal to give them more surface area to roast. Remember that 'bite-sized' for an onion usually means just chopping them into wedges; they'll soften up, the layers will separate and the slivers will shrink a little as they roast.

3. Toss all the vegetables together with the oil and a generous amount of salt and pepper on a baking tray. Roast in the oven for 30 minutes until everything is tender.

4. Meanwhile, make the dressing by whisking together the vinegar, mustard, maple syrup and olive oil until smooth. Roughly chop the parsley.

5. Remove the veggies from the oven and toss them together with the dressing and the parsley. Serve immediately.

tip

If you're making this for two, it's is lovely served on top of some brown rice.

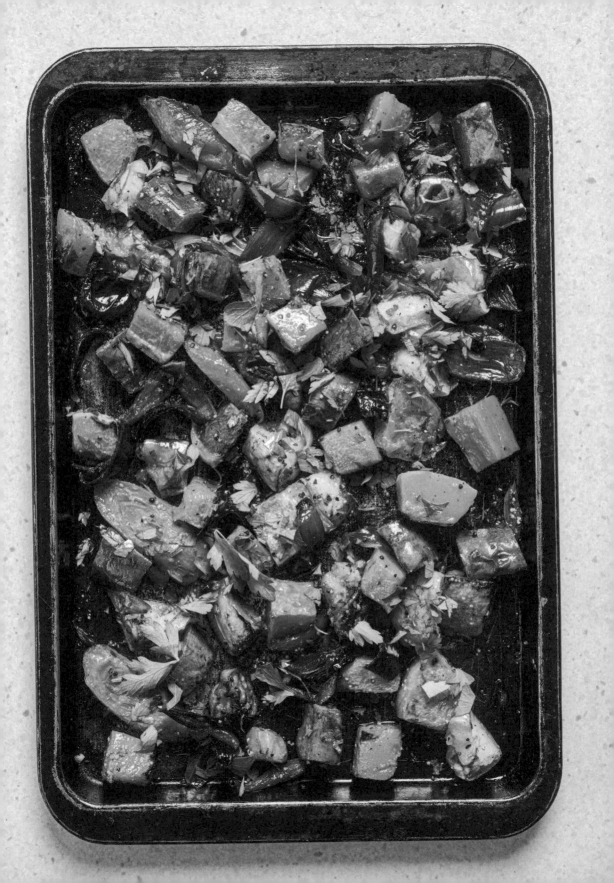

Roasted Sweet Potato and Cauliflower Hummus Bowls

SERVES 2

Preparation time: 10 minutes
Cooking time: 30–40 minutes

2 large sweet potatoes
240g (9oz) cauliflower
½ tbsp ras el hanout
1 tbsp light olive oil
1½ tbsp chermoula paste
200g (7oz) hummus (about
   1 tub)
small handful of fresh mint
large handful of pomegranate
   seeds
pomegranate or date molasses,
   for drizzling
freshly ground sea salt and black
   pepper

When I have an idea for a new recipe, I sometimes spend ages figuring out flavours in my head before I even step foot in the kitchen. However, I've spiced the cauliflower for these beautiful, Middle Eastern-inspired hummus bowls with ras el hanout and the sweet potato with chermoula because they're what I had in the cupboard the first time I made this – they just really worked well together! Feel free to experiment with your favourite Middle Eastern spices and pastes.

1. Preheat the oven to 200°C/400°F/Gas 6.

2. Cut the sweet potatoes into bite-sized cubes (don't bother peeling them) and the cauliflower into bite-sized florets.

3. Toss the cauliflower florets in one bowl along with the ras el hanout, a generous amount of salt and pepper and the olive oil until each piece is well coated. In another bowl , mix the sweet potato pieces with the chermoula and some more sea salt.

4. Spread the cauliflower out across one half of a baking sheet, and the sweet potato across the other. Roast in the oven for 30–40 minutes until the sweet potato cubes are tender and the cauliflower florets have started to char.

5. Meanwhile, divide the hummus between two shallow bowls and spread it around to create an elegant, swirled nest with the back of your spoon. Roughly chop the mint.

6. Divide the vegetables between the two bowls of hummus, and sprinkle each generously with pomegranate seeds and chopped mint. Finish each bowl with a drizzle of tangy molasses.

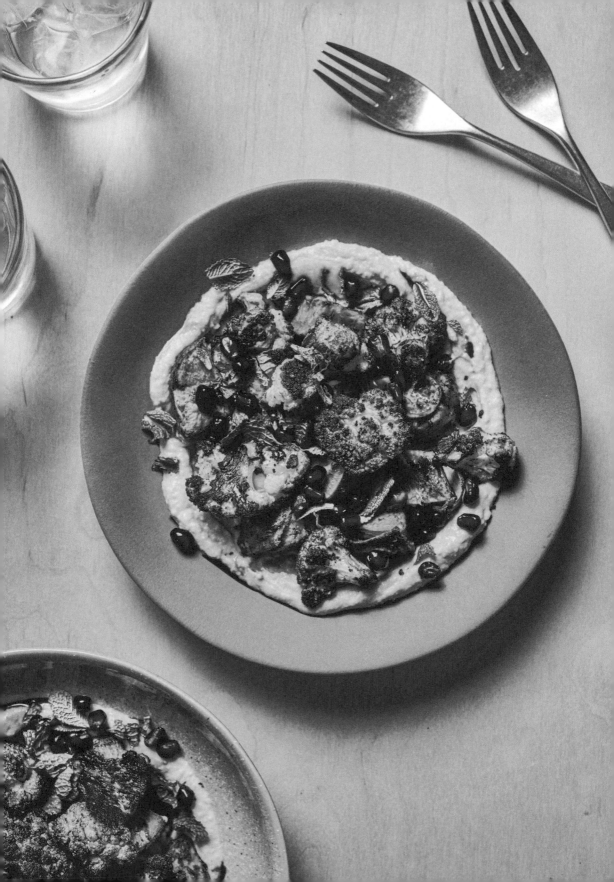

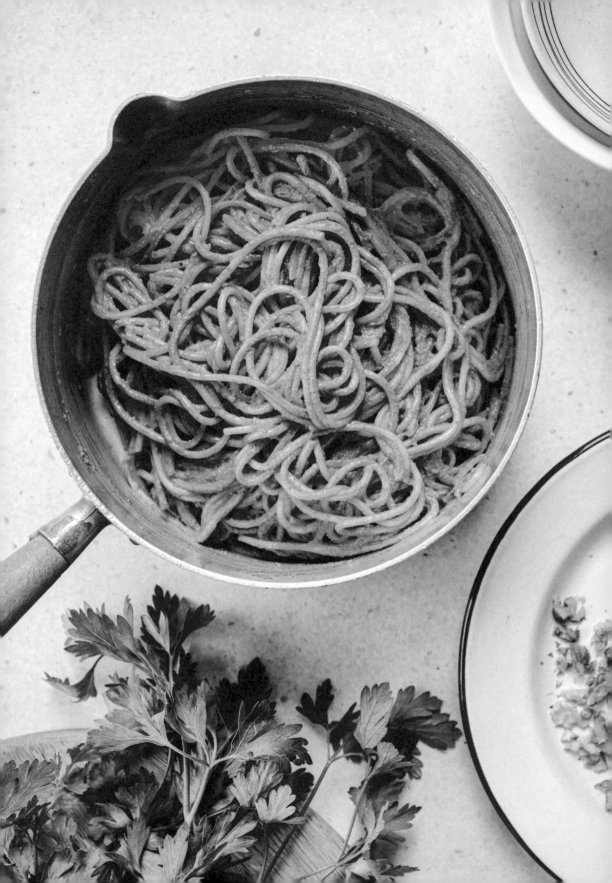

Spaghetti with Muhammara Sauce

SERVES 4

Preparation time: 5 minutes
Cooking time: 20 minutes

400g (14oz) spaghetti
20g (2 tbsp) walnut pieces
large handful of flat leaf parsley
2 batches of muhammara
  (page 42)
juice of roughly ¼ lemon, to taste

I hope I've already sold you on the wonders of muhammara, a wonderfully vibrant and flavourful red pepper and walnut dip from the Middle East (page 42). But just in case you need any more persuading, as well as being simply wonderful to scoop up pieces of toasted pitta and the odd carrot stick, muhammara also makes a fantastically bright, creamy vegan sauce for a bowl of spaghetti, with some extra chopped walnuts sprinkled on top for added crunch and a generous amount of flat leaf parsley for both colour and an extra hit of flavour.

1. Cook the spaghetti in a large saucepan of boiling salted water until the pasta is tender but still with a little bite to it; I often find the timings on the packet unreliable so start testing the odd strand after 10 minutes.

2. While the pasta is cooking, make the muhammara if you don't have it pre-made. Roughly chop the additional walnuts along with the flat leaf parsley and set aside.

3. Drain the pasta and return it to the pan. Stir in the muhammara until the pasta is bright and creamy. Divide between four warm bowls and sprinkle each with the reserved chopped walnuts, the parsley and a good squeeze of lemon juice.

Spicy, Herby
Two Pouch Mujadara

SERVES 2

Preparation time: 5 minutes
Cooking time: 45 minutes

1 large red onion

1 large white onion

3 tbsp light oil

½ tsp sea salt

½ tsp cumin seeds

½ tsp ground cinnamon

250g (9oz) pouch brown basmati rice

250g (9oz) pouch or 400g (14oz) tin green lentils in water

small handful of fresh flat leaf parsley

small handful of fresh coriander

60g (⅓ cup) pomegranate seeds

Mujadara – a gently spiced dish of rice and lentils served with caramelised onions – originated in Iraq, and is popular in different versions throughout the Middle East, especially in Jewish cuisine. I've adjusted it to my personal tastes, adding fresh herbs and jewel-like pomegranate seeds, but it is the caramelised onions that give the dish it's signature flavour – don't skimp on this slow cooking time (see tip); the rest of the dish comes together in just moments.

1. Peel the onions and use a very sharp knife to slice them into half-moons as thinly as possible.

2. Heat the oil over a medium heat in a large casserole dish or non-stick frying pan. Add the onions, sea salt and cumin seeds and gently cook for 40 minutes until the onions are soft and caramelised and have only just gone slightly brown.

3. Stir the cinnamon into the onion mixture and fry for a further minute until fragrant.

4. Break up the rice inside the pouch by gently squeezing it before opening it and tipping into the pan. If you can't find green lentils in a pouch and you're using tinned, drain these well before also adding them to the pan.

5. Stir the rice and lentils until they're well coated in the spices from the onions and heated through.

6. Taste to see if you need to add a little more salt and remove from the heat.

7. Roughly chop the herbs and stir them into the rice, along with the pomegranate seeds, just before serving.

tip

To save time you can prepare the onions ahead, store them overnight in the fridge and add them to the pan when it is time to cook – just wait until they're sizzling before you add the other ingredients.

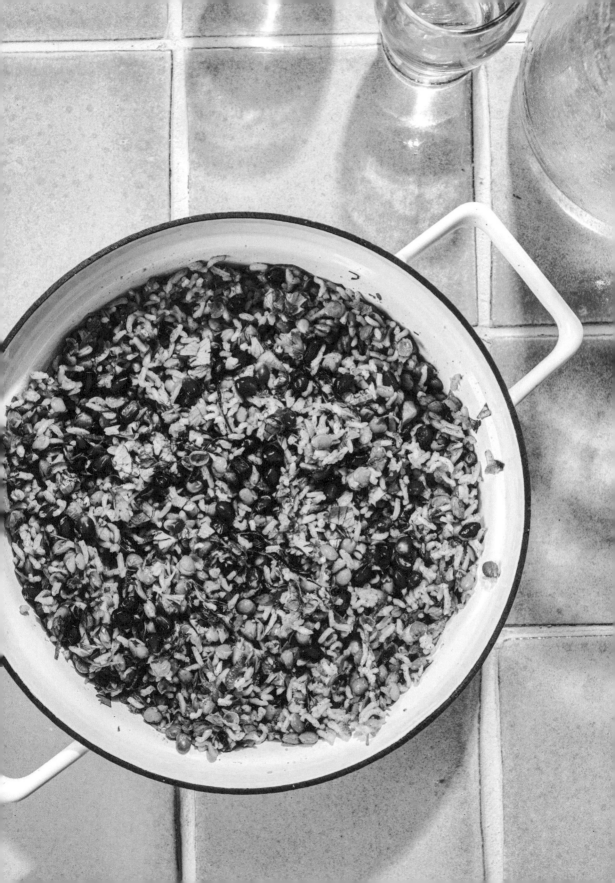

los angeles, california ——

Although I only lived there for 10 months, I don't think any single place has had as big an impact on the way I cook and eat than the city of Los Angeles. Not only is it a diverse community with a variety of rich cooking traditions that make up the Southern California's unique palate, but I challenge anyone who has been lucky enough to cook with their amazing produce and apply their unique blend of Mexican and Asian-heavy world flavours not to fall for the food of the Golden State, just one tiny bit. I fell hard.

L.A. is where I spent the second year of my degree in English Literature at the University of California, Los Angeles. It was also where — for the first time — I started to properly shop and cook for myself. I'd already cleared the first year of university living in and cooking for myself in East London, trekking down the Mile End Road on an hour-long trip to the massive Sainsbury's; but this was the time before I started shopping around in farmer's markets and greengrocers, before I had a go-to butcher and fishmonger for that little something special to supplement and enhance my day-to-day items. Before I moved to Los Angeles, fresh, seasonal ingredients that did not come in plastic were something that existed only in the country, and for some reason had not quite made it into my city cooking and the way I fed myself on a daily basis.

When I first arrived in L.A. I headed to Ralph's grocery store, in Westwood Village, which is both a wonderful and a bewildering place. Don't get me started on the frozen food aisles – there dwells all that people point to when they criticise the American diet – but when it comes to the fresh produce section at the far end of the store, that is an exciting place to be. Everything is open-plan, with big bunches of produce spilling out of the shelves and massive punnets of bright, vibrant fruit and veg piled impossibly high in big barrels in the centre of the section. It brings you a lot closer to your food in a way that can't help but make you want to load up your basket with everything fresh, green, crunchy and colourful.

I soon discovered that every Thursday at 12pm, just as I happened to be walking back from class there was a local farmer's market just a block away from my apartment. If I close my eyes now, I can see my favourite stalls and stands right in front of me. First, there was the produce stall from an upstate farm that tended to focus on heartier produce; I once bought there a big, crunchy red cabbage the size of my head which took me two weeks to eat my way through, putting away my weight in wonderfully bloody purple cabbage soups and vibrant slaws.

Next came the farm that sold the most amazing fresh berries in these lovely green, square punnets. I'd buy a trio of plump and juicy California strawberries if they had them; if not, blueberries. This is also the place I would buy my citrus fruit from; massive, knobbly lemons bigger than my hand, which I would carefully juice to make the bottles of thyme-infused lemonade

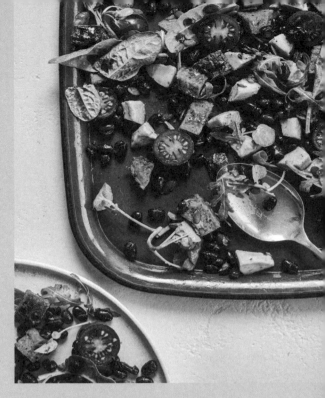

You want to load up your basket with everything fresh, green, crunchy and colourful.

I'd keep in the fridge door to glug after the hot, sweaty walk down the hill home from class. There was so much of this incredible produce, the like of which I'd never seen before; even when some of it is native to the UK, our peak seasons are nowhere as near as long as they are in the Californian sunshine.

When I returned to L.A. after university I was renting an apartment slap-bang between the Venice Canals and the beach. There, a new market became my local. Pretty much every Friday morning you could find me at Venice Farmer's Market. The fresh fruit and veg and other artisan produce on sale there blew what was available at my student market out of the water. When I visited in the spring, alongside the usual berries there were knobbly heirloom tomatoes and tiny Persian cucumbers just begging to be taken home and pickled. One seller had crates of freshly picked and unusual varieties of salad leaves for you to mix and match your own blend, as well as overflowing pots of so many different types of herbs, many of which I'd never even heard of. On my way out I'd buy a bag of beautifully chewy 'everything' bagels and a small pot of the most wonderful whipped cream cheese from the guys selling

them by the gate and a big carton of tangelo juice to enjoy for breakfast. A cross between a tangerine and a pomelo, tangelos look like slightly larger tangerines, with an intensely sweet juice that tastes somehow synthesised, like the most concentrated orange flavour created for an artificial sweet but still with an unmistakably all-natural, fresh flavour. It was at Venice Farmer's Market that I also brought home my first Meyer lemon; you can sometimes find these in London – I've spied them in Whole Foods and at Borough Market – but at an impossibly hefty price. Again, they taste unreal, like much sweeter lemons, but with the most wonderful sherbet aftertaste. While nothing will get me more excited than slicing open the perfect crimson-tinged blood orange during the gloom of midwinter in my shadowy London kitchen, for me, remembering California, there will always be that vague feeling that I'm making do.

California Kale, Orange, Almond and Mushroom Salad

SERVES 4

Preparation time: 15 minutes
Cooking time: 5 minutes

2 small banana shallots
2 tbsp rice wine vinegar
2 tsp toasted sesame oil
2 tsp maple syrup
2 tsp light olive oil
1 tsp soy sauce
8 large oranges
300g (10oz) chestnut
  mushrooms
300g (10oz) curly kale
80g (¾ cup) flaked almonds

There is a chain of healthy food canteens in California called Lemonade that do the most incredible fruit-flavoured lemonades (the guava flavour is out of this world), rainbow salads and some of the best slow cooked brisket I've ever had. My favourite Lemonade dish is their kale, orange and mushroom salad. It took me a while, but I've managed to recreate it at home, adding toasted almonds for extra crunch and to further invoke the taste of California.

1. To make the dressing, peel and thinly slice the shallots. Stir into a small bowl along with the rice wine vinegar, toasted sesame oil, maple syrup, olive oil and soy sauce.

2. Segment the oranges. To do this, slice a little off the top and the bottom of the orange, so you can sit the orange flat on the chopping board. Holding the orange flat, cutting downwards, slice off the skin with a sharp knife, working clockwise. Turn the orange over and trim off any excess skin and pith. Then, gently remove the orange segments by gently slicing either side of the membrane to release the slivers of flesh. Roughly chop the segments and add them to the bowl. It is tempting to include the juice from the chopping board to the dressing, but resist: this will make your salad too wet.

3. Halve the mushrooms down the middle then slice each half very thinly. Add the mushroom slices to the dressing, and stir so they are well coated. Set aside.

4. Roughly chop the kale, removing the tough stems, and transfer it to a large bowl. If you're using pre-chopped kale, I tend to pick out pieces of stalk as I measure the kale into the bowl.

This salad is great to make ahead, as the kale holds up to sitting in the dressing in a way that regular salad leaves never do.

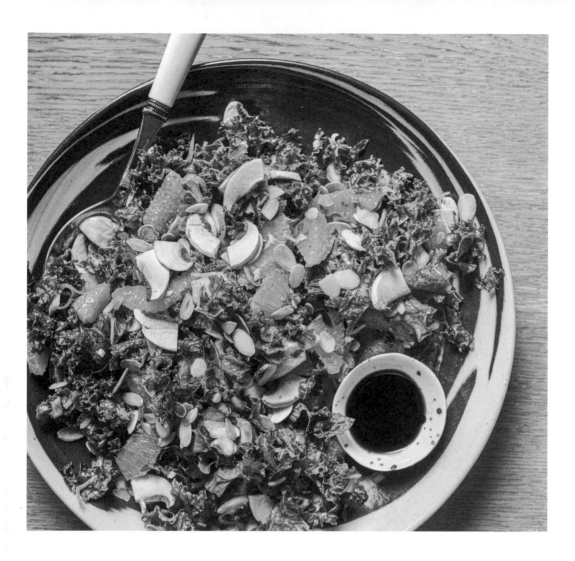

5. Massage the kale until it is soft and starting to turn your hands damp and green. I do this by rubbing the kale between my thumb and fingertips, much like rubbing butter into flour to make pastry.

6. Pour the dressing on to the kale and stir so that the kale is well coated; I find this easiest to do with my hands before I wash off all the green!

7. Put the almonds into a small frying pan over a medium-high heat and toss every minute or so until they're just going golden. Keep an eye on them – they'll go from toasted to burnt really quickly! Stir the almonds into the salad just before serving.

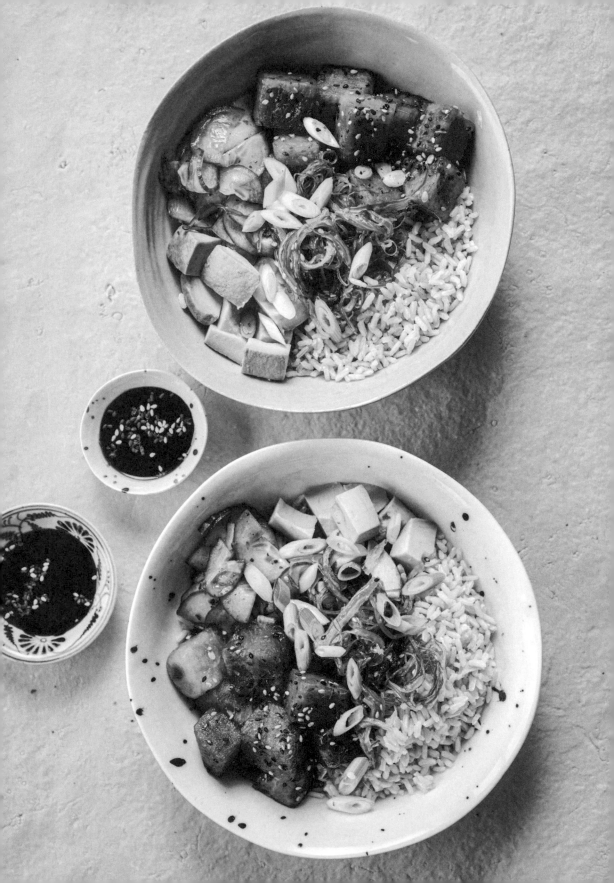

Vegan Watermelon Poke Bowls

SERVES 2

Preparation time: 10 minutes
Cooking time: 20 minutes

110g (½ cup) brown basmati rice
1 avocado
2 large spring onions
80g (3oz) wakame seaweed
  salad

**For the Korean
cucumber pickles**
½ cucumber
large pinch of sea salt
½ tsp gochugaru (Korean chilli
  flakes)
½ tsp rice wine vinegar
½ tsp toasted sesame oil
¼ tsp golden caster sugar

For the watermelon poke
½ tbsp soy sauce
½ tbsp rice wine vinegar
½ tbsp toasted sesame oil
½ tbsp lime juice
1 tsp furikake (*make sure you use
  a vegan version if this matters
  to you*), plus extra for sprinkling
400–450g (2½ cups) cubed
  watermelon

I've fallen head over heels with this vegan poke bowl. The juicy cubes of watermelon flesh hold up beautifully to the traditional soy and rice vinegar dressing, absorbing just enough of it to take on the flavour, while remaining crunchy and mouth-watering in the middle. You can serve this with any toppings you wish – check out my **Easy Salmon Poke Bowl** on page 164 for inspiration – but I think this works beautifully with quick pickled kimchee-style cucumbers, cubes of creamy avocado and lots of spring onion.

1. First cook the rice in a saucepan of boiling water for 20 minutes until tender. Drain and set aside to cool. If you're on a tight deadline, you can always cool it under the cold tap, but be sure to drain it really, really well to avoid soggy poke!

2. Meanwhile, prepare your toppings. Peel and cube the avocado and top, tail and thinly slice the spring onions.

3. To make the Korean cucumber pickles, split the cucumber down the middle lengthways – don't bother peeling it. Thinly slice the cucumber halves into half-moons and transfer to a small bowl. Add the rest of the ingredients and stir well so that the cucumber is coated in the spicy brine.

4. To make the watermelon poke, whisk together the soy sauce, rice wine vinegar, sesame oil, lime juice and furikake and then toss through the watermelon cubes. Set aside.

5. To assemble your poke bowls, arrange all of the ingredients over the top of the rice, divided between two bowls, finishing with an extra sprinkle of furikake. You'll have a lot of excess liquid leftover from making the cucumber pickles and the watermelon poke; discard the former, but the latter is delicious, as required, spooned over the bowl as extra dressing.

Sweet Chilli and Pepper Barbecue Tofu Skewers

SERVES 4

Preparation time: 10 minutes
Cooking time: 20 minutes

300g (10oz) extra firm tofu
1 tsp Chinese five spice
1 tsp garlic granules
2 red peppers
2 yellow peppers
2 red onions
160ml (⅔ cup) sweet chilli sauce
2 tbsp soy sauce
2 tbsp rice wine vinegar

I think vegetarians have, in the past, been given the short straw at barbecues and other outdoor grilling occasions. This is how I came to create a barbecue skewer that I – as a meat eater – think tastes really great, but is totally plant-based.

1. Get the barbecue ready to cook. You want a nice, steady heat in the middle, with a slightly cooler area around the edge to move skewers off into if a bit too much marinade drips down on to the coals; this will create flame, which creates smoke, which will make your food taste bad!

2. Cut the tofu into large cubes, patting dry with kitchen paper to remove as much excess moisture as possible. Put the cubes into a bowl with the five spice and the garlic granules and toss until well coated, then set aside.

3. Deseed the peppers and peel the onions. Cut everything into manageable, bite-sized chunks.

4. Alternately thread the tofu cubes, different coloured peppers and onion wedges on to the skewers, making sure not to be too rough with the tofu in case it falls apart, and not to leave a tofu cube on the end of the skewer without something to secure it for much the same reason.

5. Whisk together the sweet chilli sauce, soy sauce and rice wine vinegar to make the glaze.

tip

Soak your wooden barbecue skewers in water before assembly to stop them catching light when you're grilling.

6. Brush each skewer with the glaze and set to cook on the barbecue for 15–20 minutes until the peppers and onions are soft, and everything has just started to char, brushing the skewers with the glaze until you run out.

Deli Counter Hummus Pasta

SERVES 2

Preparation time: 10 minutes
Cooking time: 20 minutes

200g (7oz) pasta shapes
150g (¾ cup) cherry tomatoes
100g (3½oz) jarred roasted
  peppers
80g (1⅓oz) sun-dried or
  sun-blush tomatoes
60g (⅓ cup) black olives
6 tbsp hummus
juice of roughly ½ lemon
freshly ground sea salt and black
  pepper
handful of fresh basil

This is one of those storecupboard pasta dishes that is perfect to make if you need to produce a quick and easy lunch or dinner when you've forgotten to go food shopping; you just need a half-eaten tub of hummus and any leftovers that were meant to go in salads, on pizzas or to be enjoyed as antipasti that you have hanging around in your fridge. My mother is forever lamenting about how I seem to populate every fridge I have access to with jars of things, but here that sort of behaviour is helpful!

1. Cook the pasta in a saucepan of boiling salted water as per the packet instructions. I find that cooking times can be unreliable so start testing the odd piece after 10 minutes.

2. Meanwhile, quarter the cherry tomatoes and roughly chop the peppers into bite-sized pieces, making sure to pat them dry of any excess preserving liquid on a piece of kitchen paper as you go. Do the same with the preserved tomatoes. Halve or quarter the olives depending on their size.

3. Drain the pasta and stir in the vegetables and hummus until the hummus has coated the pasta. Season to taste with lemon juice, salt and pepper and serve topped with torn basil leaves.

tip

If you don't have cherry tomatoes don't worry – just increase the amount of the preserved peppers and preserved tomatoes instead.

Roast Aubergine and Fresh Tomato Salad with Basil Vinaigrette

SERVES 1–2

Preparation time: 10 minutes
Cooking time: 20 minutes

1 large aubergine
1 tbsp extra virgin olive oil
½ tsp coriander seeds
150–200g (5–7oz) mixed
  tomatoes
coconut yogurt (for drizzling)
25g (2½ tbsp) pomegranate
  seeds
freshly ground sea salt and black
  pepper

For the basil vinaigrette
1 small garlic clove
small handful of fresh flat leaf
  parsley
small handful of fresh basil
pinch of sea salt
1 tbsp white balsamic vinegar
3 tbsp extra virgin olive oil

tip

If you have any dressing left over you can store it in a jar in the fridge to use on other salads, it will keep for up to a week.

One late September lunchtime I was hungry and didn't fancy anything in my fridge so I set off down the high street in search of lunch. Some big, bulbous shiny aubergines and a massive tray of tomatoes took my fancy outside the greengrocers and fishmongers respectively, and, together with some basil (I usually keep a pot on my kitchen table) blitzed into a quick vinaigrette, they made for a really colourful, satisfying last-minute lunch.

1. Preheat the oven to 200°C/400°F/Gas 6. Roughly chop the aubergine into approximately 3cm (1¼in) cubes, and toss together with the olive oil, a generous amount of sea salt and black pepper and the coriander seeds, crushed slightly between your fingertips, on a baking tray. Roast in the oven for 20 minutes.

2. To make the basil vinaigrette, combine the garlic, herbs, sea salt and vinegar together in a small mini chopper or food processor along with 1 tablespoon of the olive oil. Blitz until smooth. You want to use as little oil as possible as there will be a lot absorbed into the aubergine and some food processors can do a nice dressing with just one spoonful, but you'll still get a great salad adding up to 2 tablespoons if you need to add more!

3. Roughly chop the tomatoes so they're about the same size as the aubergine chunks.

4. Scatter the hot aubergine on a salad plate with the cold tomato. Add generous dollops of coconut yogurt around the plate before drizzling with the vinaigrette and sprinkling with pomegranate seeds. Serve immediately.

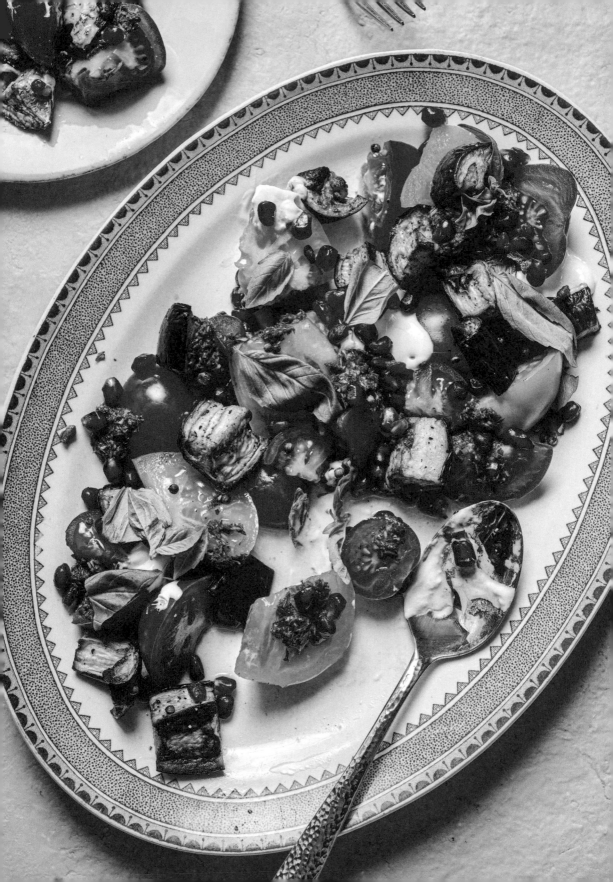

Hummus Toast with Tomatoes, Chickpeas and Crispy Kale

SERVES 2

Preparation time: 5 minutes
Cooking time: 20 minutes

300g (1½ cups) cherry tomatoes
extra virgin olive oil, for drizzling
200g (1¼ cups) chickpeas, from a
    tin or jar
2 tsp balsamic vinegar, plus extra
    for drizzling
50g (2oz) curly kale
large pinch of sea salt
2 thick slices of sourdough bread,
    toasted
4–6 tbsp hummus

This recipe started life as a brunch idea on my blog, but I've kept on tweaking it over the years and I now regularly make it as a fridge-clearing lunch option. Kale is beautiful when you roast it – still soft in the middle, but with nice crispy curls around the outside, adding texture as well as a beautiful earthy green colour to the plate. Chickpeas also transform from soft tender balls to savoury, crunchy nuggets that add a whole new type of texture to any dish.

1. Preheat the oven to 200°C/400°F/Gas 6. Halve the cherry tomatoes and spread them out, cut side up, across one-third of a large baking tray and drizzle with a little olive oil.

2. Drain and gently pat the chickpeas dry on a piece of kitchen paper and toss in a small bowl with the balsamic vinegar. Spread them out across another third of the baking tray and transfer to the oven to roast for 10 minutes.

3. Meanwhile, massage the kale with a large pinch of sea salt until it is soft and slightly damp. I do this in a large bowl using a similar motion to when rubbing butter into flour to make pastry. If I'm using a bag of pre-chopped kale, I go through and pick out all of the particularly thick and tough pieces of stalk first.

4. Remove the baking tray from the oven, toss the massaged kale with another drizzle of oil and spread it out across the remaining third of the tray. Roast for another 5 minutes until the kale has started to go crisp and golden around the edges.

5. Slather the top of each slice of sourdough toast with a thick layer of hummus before piling on first the tomatoes, then the chickpeas, then the kale. Finish with another drizzle of olive oil and balsamic vinegar, and another sprinkle of sea salt.

Tomato Salad with Pomegranate Molasses

SERVES 2
(OR 4 AS A SIDE)

Preparation time: 10 minutes
Cooking time: 40 minutes

200g (1 cup) cherry tomatoes
1 tbsp extra virgin olive oil, plus
    extra for drizzling
400–450g (14–16oz) heirloom
    tomatoes
small handful of sage flowers
    (*fresh oregano or thyme leaves
    would also work*)
pomegranate molasses, for
    drizzling
flaky sea salt (*preferably fleur de
    sel*)

While my everyday salads are usually just simply dressed with a slug of good olive oil and some of my favourite Breton *fleur de sel* salt– and maybe some fresh herbs if I'm in the mood – this salad is something a bit special. By slowly roasting the cherry tomatoes you add some beautiful, caramelised depth, and pomegranate molasses behaves a lot like balsamic vinegar when you drizzle it over fresh fruit and veg.

1. Preheat the oven to 120°C/250°F/Gas ½. Halve the cherry tomatoes and place them cut side up on a baking tray. Drizzle with a tablespoon of olive oil, transfer to the oven and roast for 40 minutes.

2. Meanwhile, slice the heirloom tomatoes into beautiful round discs and lay them – alternating colours if you've got a mixed bunch – across a large serving platter. Sprinkle with a good amount of sea salt and set aside to let the salt bring the flavours and the juices out of the tomatoes. If you're using fresh thyme, which is a bit more robust for soaking than sage flowers or fresh oregano, sprinkle that over the salad now to allow the thyme flavour to also infuse into the tomato juices.

3. Season the cooked cherry tomatoes with a little more sea salt before scattering them over the salad plate along with the sage flowers or fresh oregano leaves. Drizzle with a little pomegranate molasses before serving.

tip

Using sage flowers instead of the woodier leaves allows you to add the flavour of the herb to something that would normally be texturally unsuited to it.

Plantain Tacos with Quick Pickled Onions and Smashed Avocado

SERVES 4

Preparation time: 10 minutes
Cooking time: 20 minutes

4 ripe plantains
2 tsp light oil
1 tsp hot smoked paprika
1 small red onion
1 tbsp cider vinegar
2 large ripe avocados
fresh lime juice
12 fresh corn or soft flour taco
   tortillas
sea salt

Plantains – those funny things outside some greengrocers that look like fat bananas – are a pretty new ingredient for me. After first ordering them, fried, in a Caribbean restaurant in Notting Hill I experimented a bit and found they were equally delicious spiced and baked. I always love trying tacos with new fillings, which is how I came up with this weird and wonderful recipe. The paprika-spiced roasted plantains, combined with quick pickled onions and a good dollop of creamy smashed avocado, make for a truly satisfying result.

1. Preheat the oven to 180°C/350°F/Gas 4. Peel and thickly slice the plantain on the diagonal and toss on to a baking tray along with the oil, paprika and a good pinch of salt. Bake in the oven for 20 minutes, turning the plantain over halfway through to crisp on each side.

2. Meanwhile, peel and thinly slice the red onion and combine in a small bowl with the cider vinegar and 1 tablespoon of cold water. Set aside.

3. Peel the avocados and in a small bowl roughly mash with a fork before seasoning to taste with sea salt and lime juice. I like to go guacamole-style here – smooth, but still with some distinct chunks. Set aside.

4. Just as you take the plantain out of the oven, drain the pickled onions and pat them dry on a piece of kitchen roll.

5. Gently warm the tortillas (depending on the brand you buy they may need toasting in a blisteringly hot frying pan) and serve each piled with a couple of pieces of plantain, a couple of pickled onions and a generous dollop of avocado.

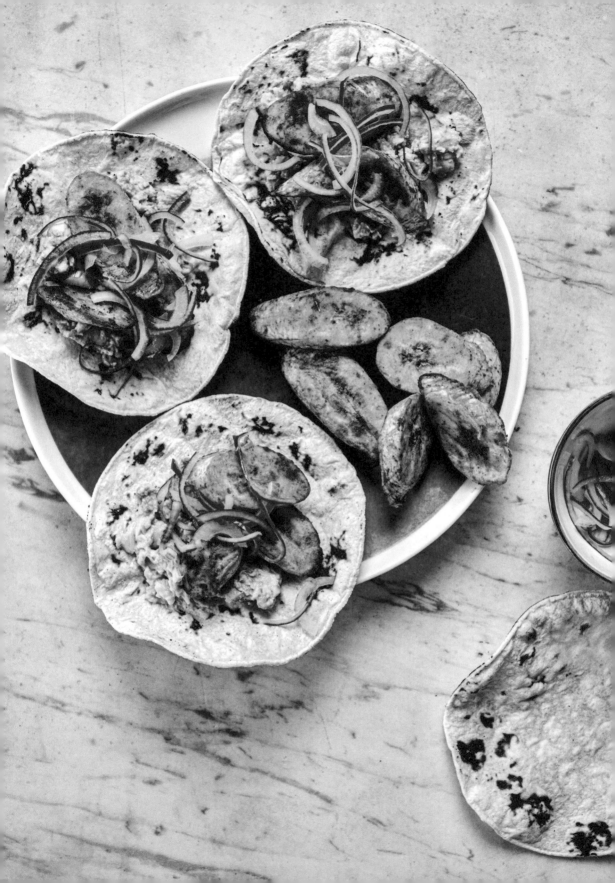

Tex-Mex Tofu Scramble

SERVES 2

Preparation time: 5 minutes
Cooking time: 5 minutes

generous glug of light oil
150g (2½ cups) tinned black
  beans
10 tbsp fresh salsa, plus extra to
  serve
200g (7oz) silken tofu
½ tsp ground turmeric
½ tsp garlic granules
freshly ground sea salt and black
  pepper

To serve
handful of freshly chopped
  coriander
1 large avocado, sliced
2 toasted tortilla wraps
hot sauce of your choice
  (*optional*)

I didn't think I would enjoy a tofu scramble as much as scrambled eggs. However, I hate food waste and one day I had some tofu left over from making my **Slow Cooker Ramen** (page 85) and searched for tofu scramble recipes instead. I flavoured the tofu with turmeric (for colour as well as taste) and garlic granules. Then, as I would do with eggs, finished the whole thing off with black beans and doused the tortillas with hot sauce just before serving.

1. Heat the oil in a non-stick frying pan over a medium heat. Add the beans and the salsa, stir to combine and heat until the mixture is starting to sizzle.

2. Drain the tofu and gently mash it with a fork. You want it to still have a few chunks, just think about the texture of regular scrambled eggs.

3. Stir the tofu into the bean mixture. Sprinkle over the turmeric, garlic granules and a generous amount of salt and pepper and stir until everything is combined and the tofu is uniform in colour. Be sure not to over stir and break up the tofu so much that it turns to mush.

4. Heat the tofu through, and serve immediately in a warm bowl. Sprinkle with coriander and serve with sliced avocado and warm tortillas, doused in hot sauce.

Creamy Sweetcorn and Chipotle Soup

SERVES 2

Preparation time: 10 minutes
Cooking time: 35 minutes

light oil, for frying
1 small onion
1 large garlic clove
1 potato
½ tbsp chipotle paste
2 large corn on the cobs
550ml (2⅓ cups) vegetable stock
sea salt

This Mexican-inspired creamy and wholesome soup comes from two very distinct places. First, while I never buy pre-made soups I spied something similar in the chilled section of Whole Foods and I was quite charmed by the concept. Secondly, I'm an avid reader of the American food website Food 52, and earlier this year they ran a piece about how you can simmer the leftover husks from corn on the cob to make a rich, corn-flavoured broth.

1. Heat a splash of oil in a large saucepan over a medium-high heat. Peel and roughly chop the onion before adding it to the pan along with a large pinch of sea salt and gently fry for 5 minutes or so until it is soft and just starting to brown around the edges.

2. Peel and crush the garlic, add to the pan and fry for a further minute until soft and aromatic. Roughly chop the potato (no need to peel it) and stir it into the onions along with the chipotle paste.

3. Meanwhile, slice the corn kernels off the husks, cleaning any wisps off the cob first. Hold the cobs upright on a cutting board and use a large, sharp knife to slice off the corn, working in a sweeping downward motion and rotating the cob as you go.

4. Add the husks to the pan along with the stock. Turn up the heat and bring the pan to the boil, then reduce the heat to medium-low and allow to simmer for 15 minutes.

5. Add the corn kernels and allow the soup to simmer for 10 minutes more until the corn is tender.

6. Using a pair of tongs, fish out and discard the corn husks. Using a hand-held blender process the soup until smooth, then check to see if you'd like to add a little more salt before serving.

tip

You can serve this plain, with a spritz of lime juice on top or, if you're not following a totally plant-based diet, a good dollop of soured cream.

Slow Cooker Mixed Bean Chilli

SERVES 2–4

Preparation time: 10 minutes
Cooking time: 3–6 hours

2 white onions
1½ yellow peppers
½ tbsp light oil (*optional, see step 2*)
400g (14oz) tin mixed beans
400g (14oz) tin black beans
400g (14oz) tin chopped tomatoes
1½ tbsp Cajun spice mix
1 tsp cocoa powder
½ tsp ground cumin

I've been making a version of a Cajun-spiced mixed bean chilli since I was a student. It started life in the big old battered saucepan that I inherited from my aunt's student digs, but now is my favourite thing to make in the slow cooker. I was resistant to getting one for ages, so used to the warming oven of the Aga I grew up cooking on, but I'm now more than slightly in love with using it to make tender curries, slow-cooked spiced meats to stuff into tacos and burritos, and to make homemade stock (recipe on page 99).

1. Peel the onions and deseed the peppers before cutting them into bite-sized chunks.

2. You'll get a delicious chilli regardless but if, like me, you have a slow cooker with one of those removable metal inserts you can heat directly over a gas hob (some electric, non-induction hobs also allow this treatment), you can add a lovely smokiness by heating ½ tablespoon of light oil in it over a high heat, and quickly frying the peppers and onions for 5 minutes until they have just started to soften and char.

3. Drain and rinse the beans and add them, along with the rest of the ingredients, to the slow cooker. Stir until everything is well combined, and cook for 3 hours on high, or 6 hours on low before serving with your favourite accompaniments.

tip

Serve with your ideal combination of grated cheese, soured cream, coconut yogurt, avocado, guacamole, salsa, tortilla chips or fresh coriander.

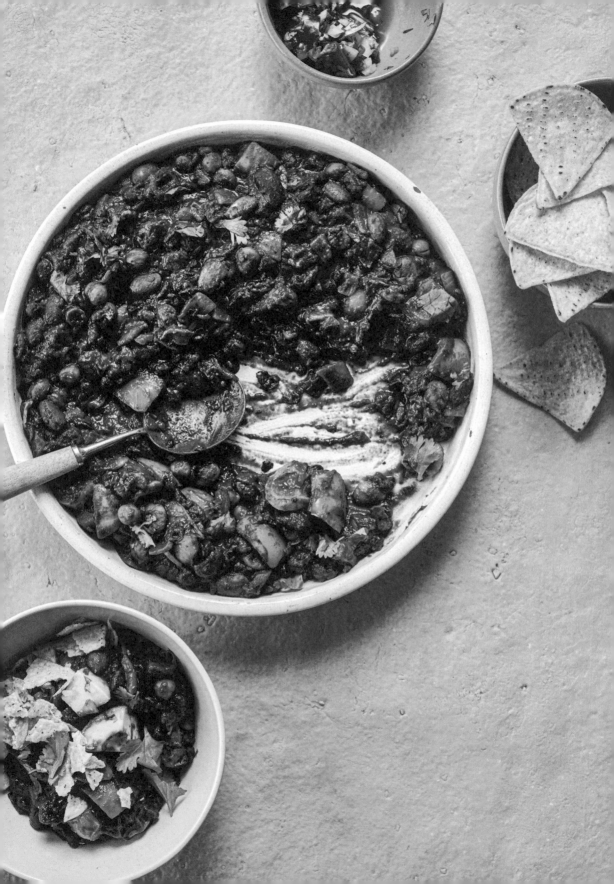

Sheet Pan Chickpea Fajitas

SERVES 2

Preparation time: 10 minutes
Cooking time: 20 minutes

1 red pepper
1 orange or yellow pepper
1 large white onion
400g (14oz) tin chickpeas
1 tsp chilli powder
¼ tsp ground cumin
¼ tsp sweet paprika
¼ tsp dried oregano
pinch of sea salt
2 tsp light oil
juice of ½ lime

To serve
4–6 flour tortillas
soured cream or coconut yogurt
fresh salsa
guacamole

Homemade fajitas are one of my favourite weeknight suppers and something we've enjoyed as a family on Saturday nights for years. They're especially good brought to the table with a selection of different salsas, creamy sauces and a good guacamole. I used to make fajitas with chicken, steak and prawns, but it was only on an empty fridge day when I was scraping around for dinner that I discovered the total deliciousness that is a hearty fajita wrap made with crispy, crunchy and deeply spicy roasted chickpeas.

1. Preheat the oven to 200°C/400°F/Gas 6. Deseed and slice the peppers and peel and cut the onion into wedges. Spread them out across a large baking tray along with the chickpeas, rinsed and drained.

2. Combine the spices, dried oregano and sea salt with the oil and drizzle over the veggies and the chickpeas. Toss until everything is coated, and roast in the oven for 20 minutes until the chickpeas are crispy and the vegetables are soft and slightly charred.

3. Squeeze the lime juice over the tray before serving with soft flour tortillas, and your choice of soured cream or coconut yogurt, salsa and guacamole.

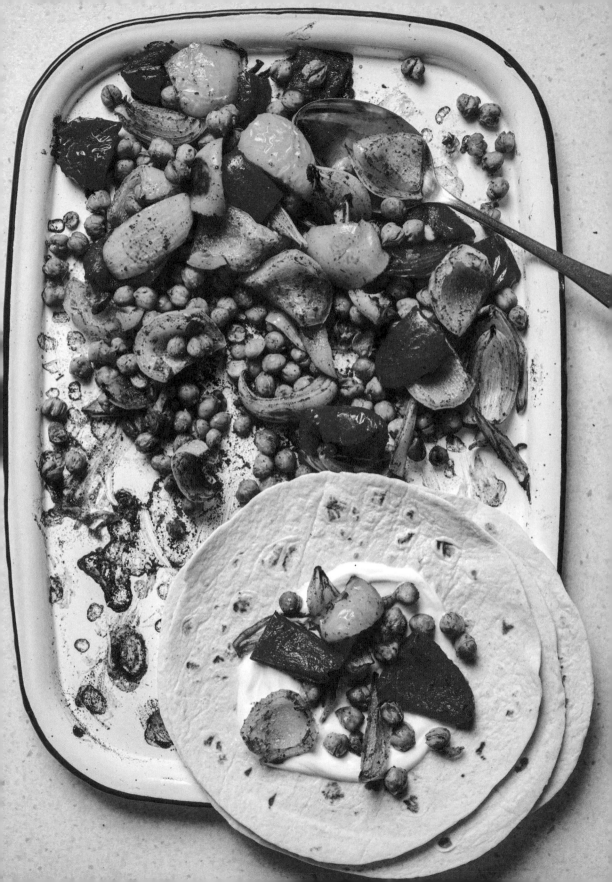

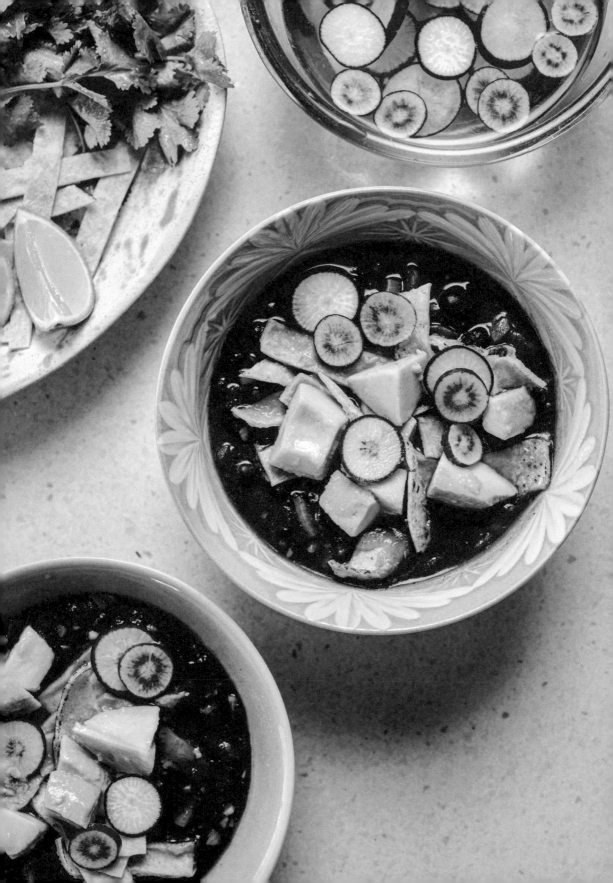

Slow Cooker Spicy Tortilla Soup

SERVES 2–3

Preparation time: 5 minutes
Cooking time: 4–8 hours

1 onion
2 large garlic cloves
1–1½ tbsp chipotle paste
    (*depending on how hot you like
    it, this soup can get spicy!*)
1 tsp ground cumin
½ tsp dried oregano
400g (14oz) tin chopped
    tomatoes
400g (14oz) tin black beans
500ml (2 cups) vegetable stock
sea salt (*optional*)
light oil (*optional; see step 1*)

To serve
large handful of fried corn or flour
    tortilla strips
Your choice of these toppings:
• avocado
• a squeeze of lime
• slices of radish
• coriander

This simplified version of the Mexico City-inspired soup is not only a cheap and easy slow cooker weeknight hero, but it is also perfect for people like me who love adding toppings to things for colour and flavour. It also helps me make sure not a single scrap from my fridge goes to waste. The name 'tortilla soup' comes from the fact it is literally a soup of fried tortilla pieces submerged in broth. What could be better?

1. Peel and finely chop the onion and the garlic. Combine with the chipotle paste, cumin and oregano, chopped tomatoes, black beans (drained) and the vegetable stock in the slow cooker. If you have one of those slow cookers with a removable 'sear-and-stew' insert, frying the onion and the garlic off first in a splash of oil will help deepen the flavour of the soup, but it is by no means a necessary step.

2. Cook for 4 hours on high or 7–8 hours on low. Check for seasoning – depending on your brand of chipotle paste you may not need any salt – before serving in small bowls with your chosen toppings.

Alphabet Minestrone Soup

SERVES 4

Preparation time: 15 minutes
Cooking time: 40 minutes

2 celery sticks
2 carrots
1 large white onion
1 tbsp olive oil
2 garlic cloves
1 tbsp tomato purée
300g (10oz) ripe tomatoes,
  diced
1 dried bay leaf
1 tsp dried thyme
800ml (3⅓ cups) vegetable
  stock
100g (3½oz) Savoy cabbage
50g (2oz) alphabet pasta shapes
freshly ground sea salt and black
  pepper

For the lemon pesto
30g (1 cup) fresh basil
2 tbsp extra virgin olive oil
1 tbsp pine nuts
zest of ¼ lemon
juice of roughly ½ lemon, to taste
sea salt, to taste

A classic minestrone is the soup I remember being fed most often as a child. Sometimes it was made with bacon and pasta shapes; sometimes it was meat-free and bulked out with the broken up pieces of spaghetti from the bottom of the elegant glass spaghetti jar. I've taken the dish back to childhood by using alphabet pasta shapes, though if you can't find any, I have found orzo makes a great substitute.

1. Top and tail the celery and peel the carrots and the onion. Finely chop all the vegetables.

2. Heat the oil in a large, lidded saucepan over a medium-high heat. Gently fry the chopped veggies until they are soft and starting to go slightly golden, but not brown. This should take at least 5 minutes. Add the garlic, peeled and crushed, and fry for a few minutes until aromatic. Stir in the tomato purée, the fresh tomatoes, bay leaf and thyme. Season well with salt and pepper.

3. Stir in the stock and bring to the boil. Reduce the heat to low, put on the lid and simmer for 20 minutes.

4. To make the pesto, combine the basil (leaves and stalks) with the olive oil, pine nuts and lemon zest in a food processor until smooth. Add half of the lemon juice at first and then add the rest if you want it to be smoother.

5. Shred the cabbage into thin ribbons, cutting out any tough, white inner stalks. Add the cabbage and the pasta shapes to the soup, and cook for a further 10 minutes with the lid on, until the pasta is just tender. Check the seasoning and serve with a pesto swirl in each bowl.

Green Pea and Lemon Pesto Pasta

SERVES 4

Preparation time: 5 minutes
Cooking time: 20 minutes

400g (14oz) pasta shapes
(*I usually use fusilli*)
250g (1⅔ cups) frozen petit pois,
  defrosted
large handful of fresh basil
large handful of walnuts
extra virgin olive oil
sea salt
juice of roughly ½ lemon

Pesto pasta has always been my last minute standby, but it's not really very exciting, unless you've taken the time to make a fresh pesto rather than reaching for the stuff in a jar. I pretty much always have a bag of frozen petit pois in the freezer for some last-minute veg, and here I've turned them into a bright, raw and vibrant lemony vegan pesto to toss through my pasta shapes. If you've got any leftovers, the pesto is also delicious spread on hot toast.

1. Cook the pasta in a large saucepan of boiling salted water according to the packet instructions – but do test it after about 10 minutes.

2. Meanwhile, in a small blender or food processor combine the peas, basil, walnuts and a drizzle of olive oil until almost smooth – you still want a bit of texture from the peas. Keep on adding olive oil, little by little, until you achieve this. Season to taste with sea salt and lemon juice.

3. Drain the pasta and stir in the pesto before serving.

the vegetable plot ————

One of my earliest 'outdoor' memories is of standing on an upturned bucket one afternoon after school, so that I could reach the workbench at the end of our family greenhouse to help my mum poke dried little peas into drainpipes full of soft compost ready to bloom into new pea plants come summer. Another memory is of battling my way through the raspberry canes in our vegetable plot, then much taller than I was, picking bowls of soft, finger-staining fruit before watching my mum turn it into jewel-like jars of her raspberry jam using her battered jam cauldron.

That greenhouse was right at the heart of my childhood summers. We filled the industrial-sized glass tunnel with different varieties of tomato, letting them grow tall and proud, and as August drew to a close and September beckoned there was always a massive glut to contend with. Because of this, I've become something of an expert in recipes that use up a ton of tomatoes, quickly and deliciously. There's nothing like the taste of a home-grown tomato, plucked fresh off the plant with the scent of their stalks in the air around you, and a smudge of that slightly sticky yellow that coats their leaves across your fingers.

Along with the tomatoes we grew cucumbers, masses of courgettes, green beans and long, yellow French beans, bunches of sweet-smelling sweet peas for the kitchen table, and — when the rabbits and pigeons didn't get them — rows of strawberries and raspberries. One year my dad planted leeks which were a massive success, but I think he put in too many for just the three of us to tackle. There was also the year we had an entire wheelbarrow full of squash that kept us going for months, and that pumpkin, which filled our extra large reinforced wheelbarrow just by itself. Now my parents have moved house we're growing much the same but the crowning glory of the whole lot is the English rhubarb. My parents have moved house with it three times but it still produces beautiful, green- and crimson-tinged stalks perfect for compotes, crumbles and, most recently, their homemade rhubarb wine. I always carry some back to London with me to bake simply with a pinch of ginger and a splash of orange juice to have for breakfast each morning over a bowl of natural yogurt with a handful of toasted pine nuts for added crunch.

Moving out to suburbia, I've taken on a patch of shared garden which, come the spring, I hope to plant up as a kitchen garden, supplying me with enough fresh produce to seriously reduce my trips to the supermarket next summer and autumn. I'm hoping it will be enough to free up a bit more of our weekly food budget to spend at the local butcher's and fishmonger's. I've already had success with my own, late-in-the-day cut-and-come-again lettuce, and while my French breakfast radishes were eaten by the pesky

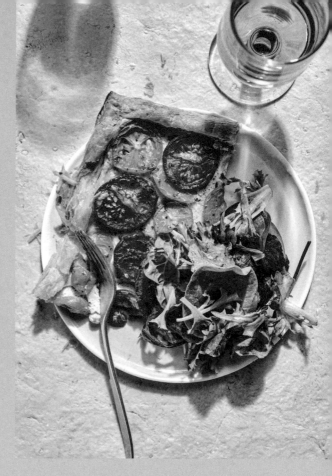

I think growing your own vegetables, even if it is just a windowsill pot of herbs, is the easiest and most rewarding way to get closer to your food.

neighbourhood squirrel, I already have chives, rosemary, mint and thyme growing on the patio, and a basil plant on the kitchen table. In an effort to cut down on kitchen waste I've also got a wormery just by the back door where my little army of worms are busy turning all our eggshells and vegetable peelings into a steady supply of all-natural compost and liquid fertiliser to feed my future efforts.

I think growing your own vegetables, even if it is just a windowsill pot of herbs, is the easiest and most rewarding way to get closer to your food, and to become more enthusiastic about predominantly plant-based eating. I know I've been very privileged, and have been raised by a family who have always done their best to grow their own, but growing something yourself to add colour and a sense of accomplishment to your meals is easier than you might think. If you look online or in garden centres, there are tons of different types of herbs and micro greens you can grow in old yogurt pots and the like which

you simply can't buy anywhere else. Cut-and-come-again lettuce is also a good windowsill crop, and you can buy a packet of seeds, a planting tray and a little bit of compost for less than £3.

If you are lucky enough to have a bit of outdoor space, go online to see people who are doing some really smart things with DIY vertical planting. If you have a little bit of a balcony (or even a hook out of a window you can safely suspend something from) think upwards with planters and hanging baskets and you'll be surprised at how easy it is to get planting.

Dukkah Spaghetti with Raw Tomato and Almond Sauce

SERVES 4

Preparation time: 5 minutes, plus
  overnight soaking time
Cooking time: 20 minutes

70g (½ cup) blanched almonds,
  soaked in a bowl of cold water
  for 10 hours or overnight
400g (14oz) wholemeal
  spaghetti
500g (1lb 2oz) tomatoes
2 tbsp extra virgin olive oil, plus
  extra for drizzling
2 large pinches of golden caster
  sugar
2 large pinches of sea salt
dukkah, for sprinkling

I came up with this method for making a creamy, vegan-friendly, no-cook tomato sauce as part of a recipe I was putting together for the Great British Chefs website. It's bright and vibrant, and one of those recipes you'll need to source the best, ripest summer tomatoes for, as well as your best virgin oil. Dukkah is an Egyptian dried dip made from a heady blend of toasted hazelnuts and spices that's designed for bread and fresh vegetables. It's available in small tubs in the spice section of most supermarkets. If you can't find it, do what I did the first time I made this recipe: use a little garlic, and serve it with torn fresh basil and grated Parmesan instead.

1. Cook the spaghetti in a large saucepan of boiling salted water as per the packet instructions (keep in mind that cooking times can vary so test it after 10 minutes).

2. Meanwhile, roughly chop the tomatoes and blitz them in a blender along with the olive oil, soaked almonds and a couple of large pinches of golden caster sugar and sea salt until completely smooth. Check the seasoning and add a little more salt, if needed.

3. Drain the spaghetti and return to the pan along with the tomato sauce, stirring until the pasta is well coated. Divide between four bowls and top each with a generous scattering of dukkah.

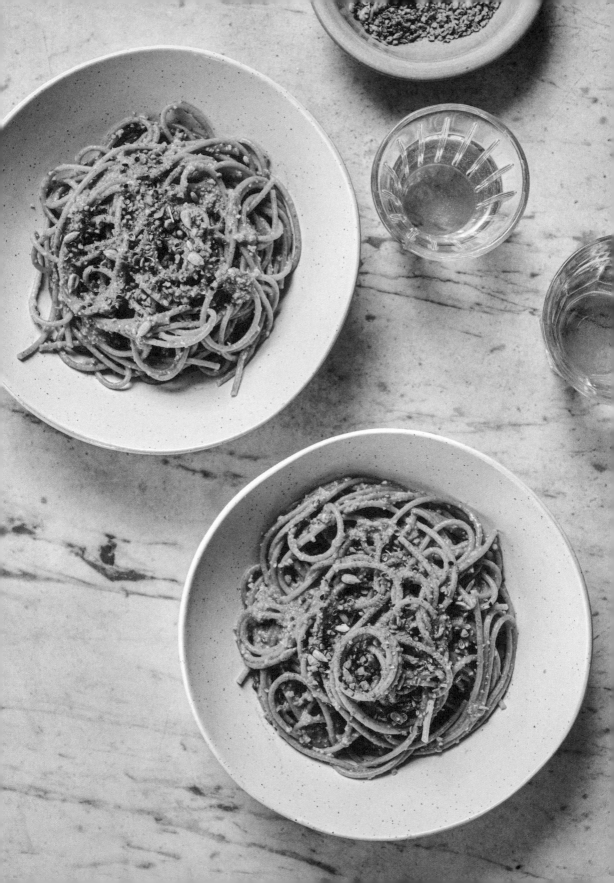

Veggie Paella

SERVES 2

Preparation time: 10 minutes
Cooking time: 40 minutes

1 onion
2 large garlic cloves
large glug of extra virgin olive oil
½ tsp hot smoked paprika
pinch of saffron strands
  (*optional*)
450ml (2 cups) vegetable stock
1 red pepper
1 yellow pepper
1 small courgette
150g (¾ cup) paella rice
2 tsp tomato purée
generous splash of white wine
200g (1 cup) cherry tomatoes
small handful of flat leaf parsley
freshly ground sea salt and black
  pepper

tip

*I find that saffron strands really
enhance the flavour of this dish so
I recommend investing in some if
you can.*

I love paella made with chicken, seafood and lots of saffron but this vegan option is a really tasty weeknight rice dish made in the same style but will take you a fraction of the time. It's got lots of tasty veggies, some smoky paprika and, while it is different to what you'll find on the streets of Spain, it is something you can achieve in under an hour on a busy weeknight. The leftovers are also delicious cold, if you're into that sort of thing.

1. Peel and chop the onion and garlic.

2. Heat a glug of oil in a large non-stick frying pan or casserole dish over a medium-high heat. Gently fry the onion until soft and starting to go golden before adding the garlic cloves. Fry for another minute until soft and aromatic, then stir in the paprika.

3. Meanwhile, steep the saffron (if using) in the vegetable stock, core and deseed the peppers and top and tail the courgette. Cut the peppers into bite-sized pieces and do the same with the courgette, cutting it down the middle first to make half-moons.

4. Add the vegetables to the pan and fry for about 5 minutes until they're starting to go soft around the edges. Add the paella rice and cook until the rice is hot before stirring in the tomato purée.

5. Add the white wine and allow that to bubble away before adding the stock, a generous amount of salt and pepper and the tomatoes. Bring the pan to the boil, then reduce to a low heat and leave to simmer without stirring for 30 minutes.

6. At this point the rice should be moist and tender without being sloppy. Check the seasoning, then serve sprinkled with roughly chopped flat leaf parsley.

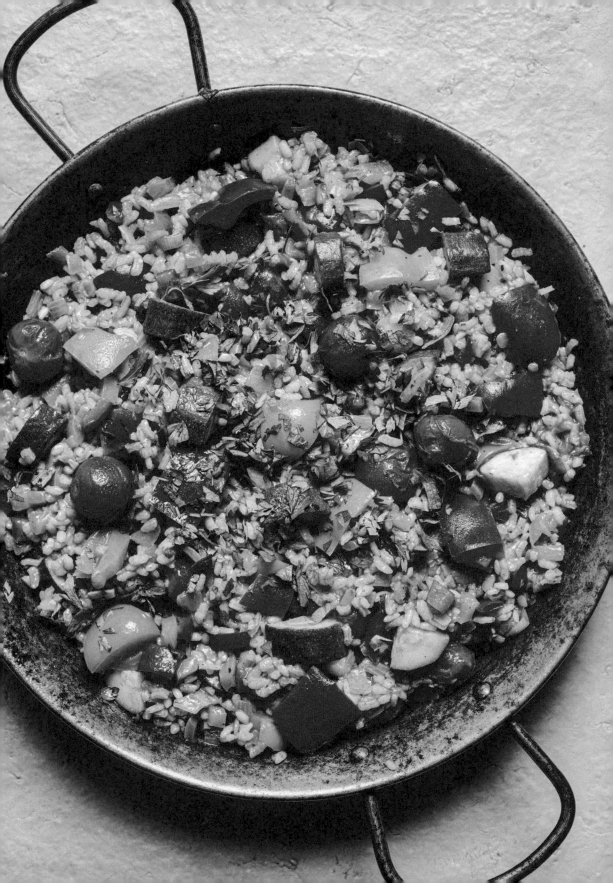

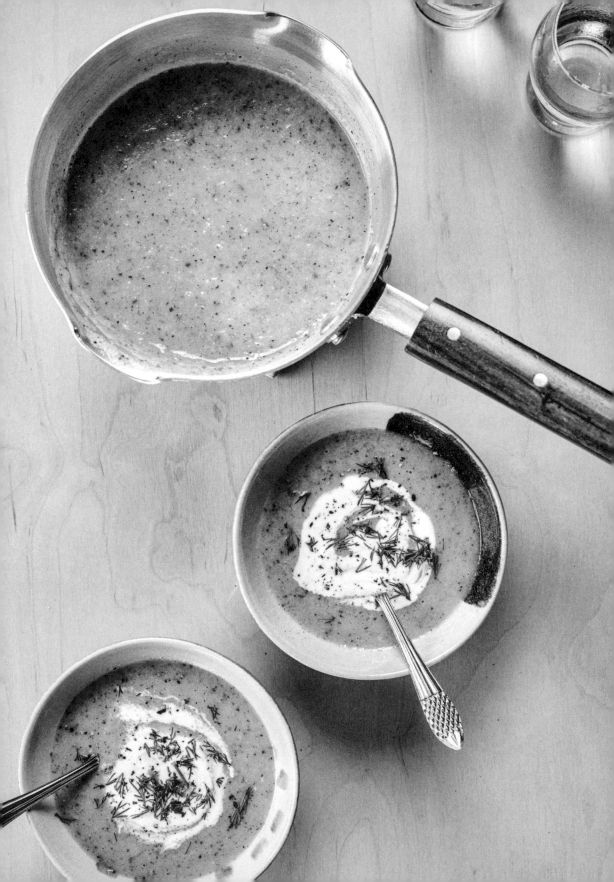

Easy Summertime Courgette Soup

SERVES 3-4

Preparation time: 15 minutes
Cooking time: 25 minutes

glug of light oil
1 white onion
1 large garlic clove
2 large courgettes
200g (7oz) potatoes
500ml (2 cups) vegetable stock
juice of roughly ¼ lemon
freshly ground sea salt and black
 pepper

To serve
natural or coconut yogurt
fresh dill

This is one of my favourite summertime soup recipes. It started life as a way for my family to get through the sheer volume of courgettes we grew every summer and it is now what I make whenever we're stuck inside on a rainy summer's day. I like to garnish this with dill, but any soft herbs from your garden or kitchen herb pots will do.

1. Heat a glug of oil in a large saucepan over a medium-high heat. Peel and roughly chop the onion and gently fry along with a good pinch of sea salt until soft and just starting to brown. Peel and crush the garlic clove, add it to the pan and fry for a further minute until fragrant.

2. Meanwhile, grate the courgettes and the potatoes (no need to peel them, just make sure they're clean) on the largest hole of the box grater.

3. Add the grated vegetables to the pan and cook for a few minutes until they're starting to soften.

4. Add the vegetable stock and a generous amount of black pepper before turning up the heat to bring to the boil. Once the broth is bubbling, turn down the heat to low and allow it to simmer for 10 minutes until the potato and courgette are tender.

5. Remove the pan from the heat and use a hand-held blender to blitz until smooth. Taste and season with more salt and pepper if needed, then add some lemon juice to add brightness and acidity.

6. Serve in warm bowls with a dollop of yogurt – natural is the easiest to find but coconut is the best vegan option, live yogurt is also particularly good here – a few sprigs of dill and another few grinds of black pepper.

Easy Ratatouille Spiral

SERVES 2–4

Preparation time: 15 minutes
Cooking time: 1 hour, plus resting
   time

2 large garlic cloves
250ml (1 cup) passata
1½ tsp golden caster sugar
1 tsp dried oregano
1 aubergine
1 courgette
3 large tomatoes
extra virgin olive oil
freshly ground sea salt and black
   pepper

This ridiculously easy baked ratatouille is a real vegan showstopper, carried to the table still in the cooking dish, perhaps sprinkled with a little fresh basil and with a warm, sliced ciabatta for mopping up the juices.

1. Preheat the oven to 200°C/400°F/Gas 6.

2. Crush the garlic cloves and mix them with the passata, sugar, oregano and a generous amount of salt and pepper in the bottom of a 22cm (9in) round baking dish. Don't worry if your dish is a few centimetres bigger or smaller – this is just how big mine is, to give you the general idea! You can also use a casserole dish or a frying pan with an ovenproof handle if you've not got one.

3. Thinly slice the aubergine, courgette and tomatoes into equal rings. To assemble the spiral, layer the vegetables around the edge of the dish, alternating between them and starting a new spiral inside the first and so on, until you've reached the middle and run out of veggies. Don't worry if it looks a bit messy – it will look far more impressive cooked than raw once the vegetables have softened and browned slightly in the oven.

4. Drizzle the spiral generously with olive oil and season again with a few more grinds of salt and pepper. Cover the dish with foil and bake in the oven for 30 minutes.

5. Take off the foil and cook for a further 30 minutes before removing from the oven.

6. Leave the spiral to rest for 5 minutes before serving to allow the juices to soak into the veggies.

tip

If you have some veggies left over I usually just roast them in the oven with some seasoning at the same time the spiral is cooking to use in salads.

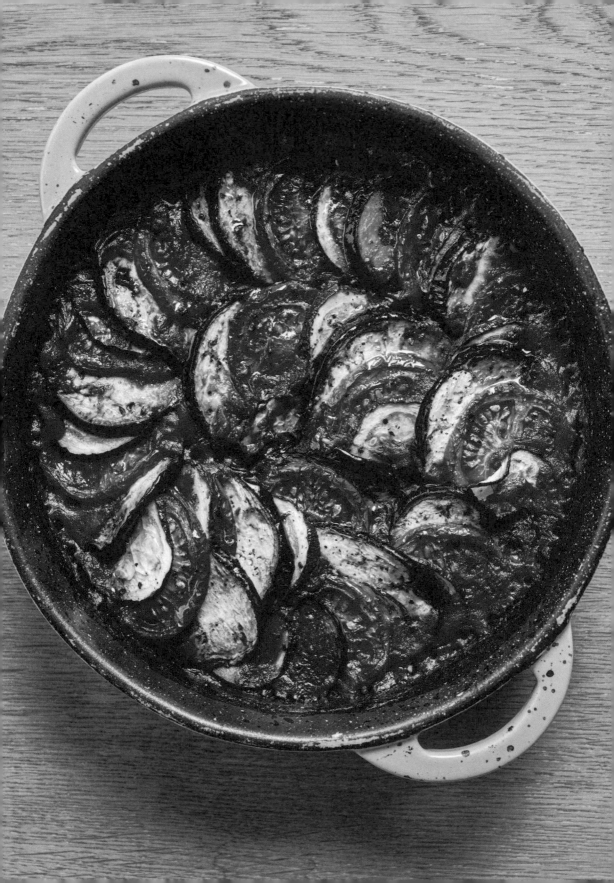

Sweet Potato Miso Soup

SERVES 4

Preparation time: 10 minutes
Cooking time: 30 minutes

generous glug of light oil, for
    frying
2 small white onions
900g (2lb) sweet potato
2 tbsp grated fresh ginger
2 pinches of dried chilli flakes
3 tbsp red miso paste
1.2 litres (5 cups) vegetable stock
4 large spring onions
sea salt (*optional*)
4 wedges fresh lime
furikake (*make sure you use
    a vegan version, if this is
    important to you*)

tip

*The reason I've used red miso
paste is simply because it was
what I had in the fridge. Each miso
will produce subtly different results
but brown and white miso paste
would make fine substitutes.*

At a Japanese restaurant in Brixton a few years ago I had a fantastic sweet potato, simply baked and split open before being filled with the most wonderful miso butter. This soup is that potato in a vegan soup form, making it perfect for a filling, nourishing autumn meal.

1. Heat a glug of oil in a large saucepan over a medium-high heat. Peel and roughly chop the onions and fry for 5–6 minutes until softened and just started to brown. Meanwhile, peel and chop the sweet potato into bite-sized cubes.

2. Add the ginger and the dried chilli flakes to the pan and fry for a further minute until aromatic.

3. Add the sweet potato chunks and the miso paste, stirring until everything is coated in the miso.

4. Add the stock and turn up the heat to bring the pan to the boil. Once it is bubbling, turn the heat down to low and allow it to simmer for roughly 25 minutes, or until the sweet potato is tender. Meanwhile, trim and thinly slice the spring onions.

5. Remove the soup from the heat and use a hand-held blender to blitz until smooth. Check the seasoning (depending on which brand of miso you're using you might want to add a touch of salt).

6. Divide the soup between four warm bowls and garnish with the spring onion slices, a good squeeze of lime – don't skimp on this, it adds important acidity to each spoonful – and a good sprinkling of furikake.

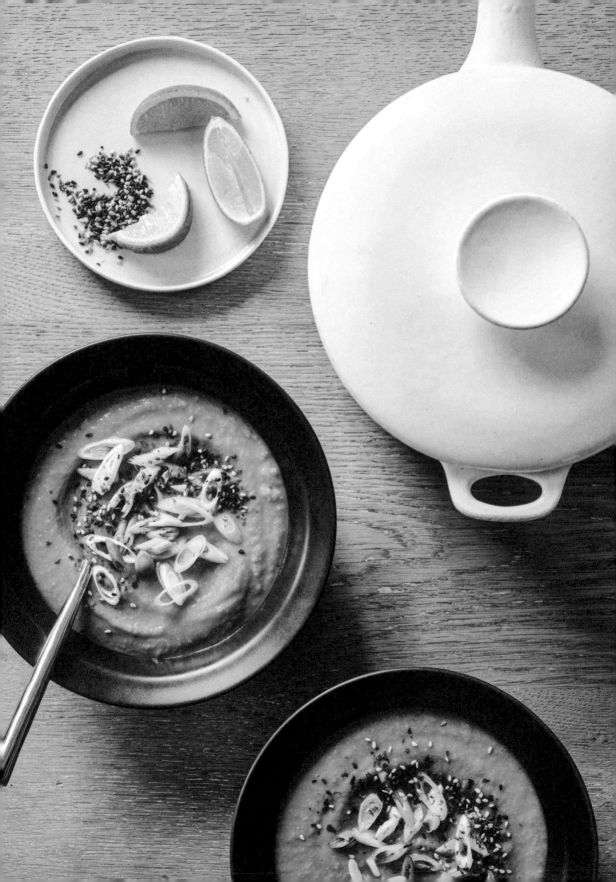

Spicy Korean Rice Cakes (*Tteokbokki*)

SERVES 1

Preparation time: 5 minutes
Cooking time: 10 minutes

4–5 large spring onions
½ courgette
4 tbsp gochujang
1 tsp soy sauce
1 tsp golden caster sugar
1 large garlic clove
250g (9oz) frozen Korean rice
  cakes, defrosted

To serve (optional)
Furikake (*make sure you
  use vegan version, if this is
  important to you*)
Kewpie mayonnaise (*note that
  this is not vegan-friendly*)

Tteokbokki, a spicy, saucy stir fry of wonderfully soft and toothsome Korean rice cakes, fish cakes and veggies, is my favourite thing to order at a Korean restaurant. I usually order it alongside a Kimchee pancake and a whole load of banchan, those small little dishes of marinated and fermented vegetables that are as important to any Korean meal as a fluffy, steaming bowl of rice. The small, cylindrical Korean rice cakes you need (not the flat oval ones) are pretty easy to find in the frozen section of most Asian supermarkets, but I find the thin, spongy, ribbon-like fish cakes almost impossible to get, so here I've created a vegan version.

1. Trim the spring onions and cut each into three short lengths. Cut the courgette (no need to peel it) into similar sized batons.

2. To make the cooking sauce, whisk together the gochujang, soy sauce, sugar and garlic clove (peeled and crushed) together with 200ml (¾ cup) water in a medium frying pan.

3. Set the pan over a high heat and bring to the boil. Reduce the heat to medium and add the rice cakes. Allow to simmer for 5 minutes, stirring occasionally, until the rice cakes begin to soften and the sauce starts to thicken.

4. Add the vegetables and cook for a further 5 minutes until the veggies are just tender and the sauce coats everything in a thick, glossy sheen.

5. Serve as is, or drizzled with a little Kewpie mayo and sprinkled with furikake.

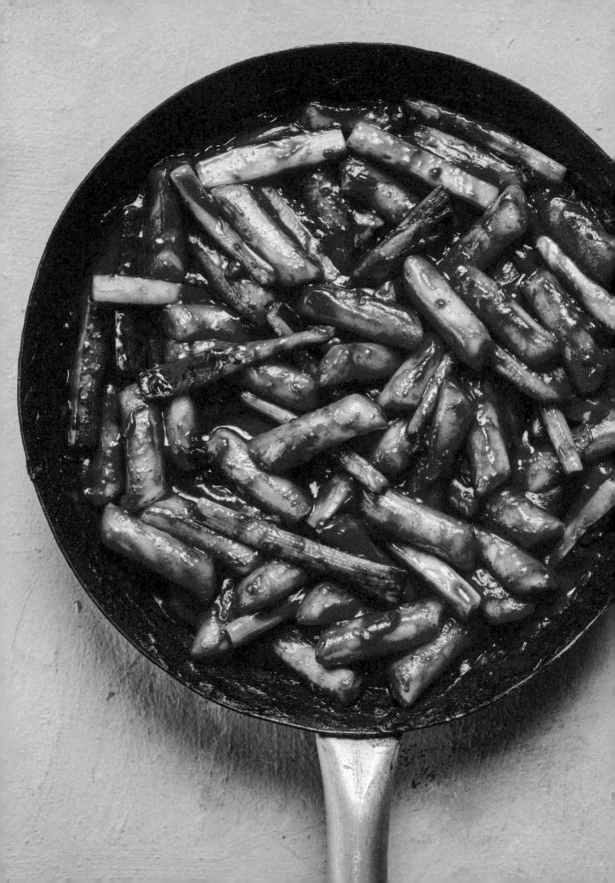

Spicy Cucumber and Silken Tofu Rice Noodles

SERVES 4

Preparation time: 5 minutes
Cooking time: 10 minutes

200g (7oz) wide rice noodles
2 cucumbers
2 × 300g (10oz) packs silken tofu
1 tbsp rice wine vinegar
2 tsp soy sauce
1 tsp golden caster sugar
1 tsp dried chilli flakes
½ tsp sea salt
large handful of fresh coriander

This quick, cold and slightly spicy noodle bowl is all about contrasts. Tender rice noodles, a chilli-flecked, vinegar-heavy sauce, crunchy cucumber and silky-soft tofu come together to make a refreshing lunch to enjoy on a hot summer's day. Rather than cutting the cucumber into half-moons, I've been known to serve it in batons, and without the noodles or tofu as a simple and refreshing side as part of an Asian-inspired feast.

1. Cook the rice noodles in a saucepan. I find that when the packet says to simply soak them in boiling water until tender it never works, so I cook them as I would egg noodles in a pan of boiling water for just a couple of minutes until they're tender. Instantly stop them from cooking further by rinsing under the cold tap; this also gets rid of the excess starch and stops them sticking together. Set aside to drain.

2. Peel the cucumbers and slice into 5mm (¼in) half-moons. Drain and carefully cut the tofu into bite-sized cubes.

3. To make the dressing, whisk together the rice wine vinegar, soy sauce, sugar, chilli flakes and sea salt.

4. Toss the dressing with the noodles along with the cucumber and coriander, roughly chopped. Carefully stir in the tofu to stop it from breaking up too much before serving.

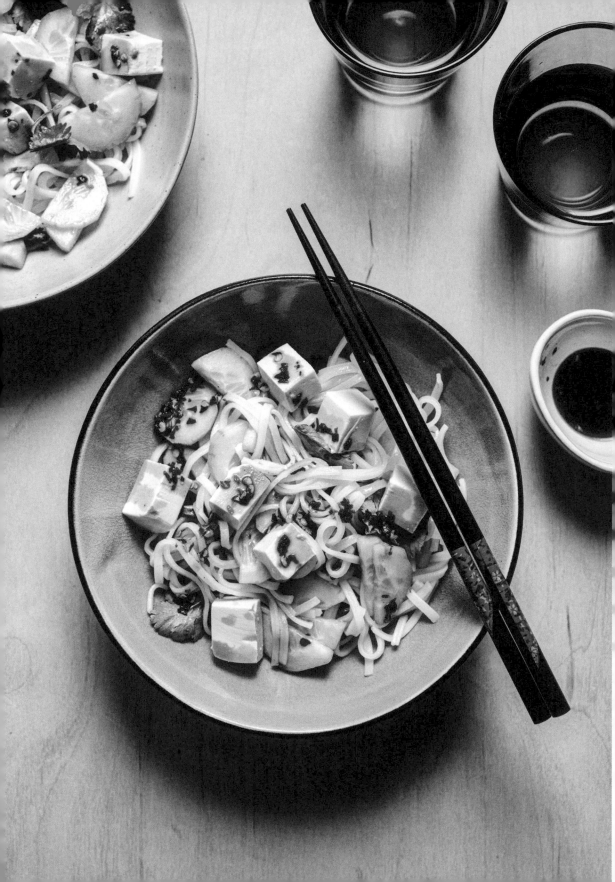

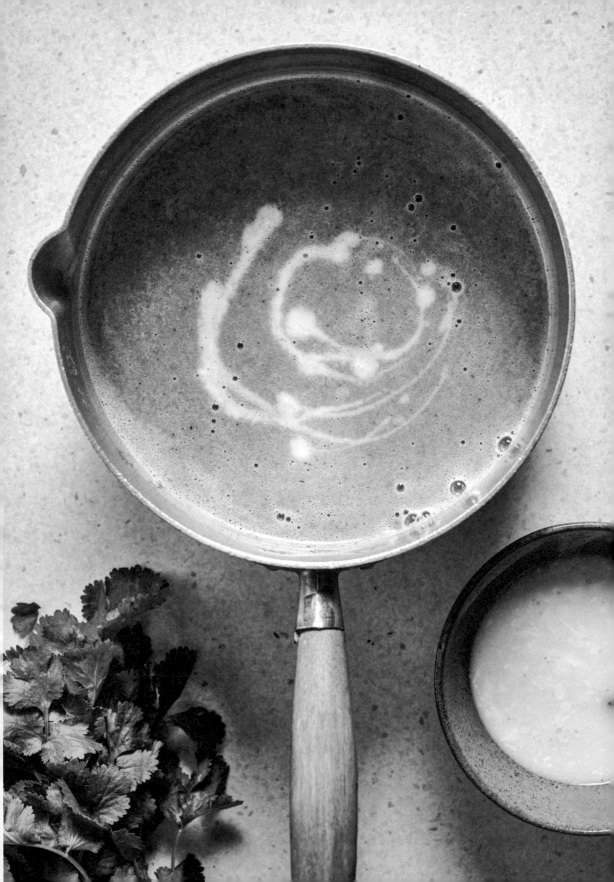

Thai Green Pea Soup

SERVES 4

Preparation time: 5 minutes
Cooking time: 15 minutes

2 tbsp vegetable oil
2 small onions
3 tbsp Thai green curry paste
600g (4 cups) frozen petit pois
1.2 litres (5 cups) vegetable stock
6 tbsp coconut milk, plus extra for
 drizzling
freshly ground sea salt and black
 pepper
fresh lime juice, to serve

This soup started life as a five-ingredient recipe for the women's lifestyle website Refinery 29. I was really proud of it – a pea soup that tasted just like a Thai green curry – what could be better? However, as is the case with a lot of recipes I create on commission but fall in love with, I kept on making it long after publication and therefore it has changed a little – I think for the better – over the course of many lunchtimes. Alas, it is no longer a five-ingredient recipe, but if, like me, you always keep a stash of homemade stock in the freezer (my recipe for **Slow Cooker Vegetable Stock** is on page 99), it is no great hardship.

1. Heat the vegetable oil in a large saucepan over a medium heat. Peel and finely chop the onions and gently fry for about 10 minutes until they are soft and only just starting to brown.

2. Add the curry paste, and fry for a further 5 minutes until aromatic.

3. Add the frozen petit pois and the vegetable stock and turn up the heat to bring to a simmer. Once the water is just starting to bubble, reduce the heat to low and allow the soup to simmer for 5 minutes until the peas have cooked through.

4. Remove the pan from the heat and blend until smooth with a hand-held blender. Blitz in the coconut milk and season to taste with salt and pepper before ladling into warm bowls. I serve each bowl with a good squeeze of lime juice for a pleasantly acidic kick in each spoonful, a good swirl of coconut milk for extra creaminess and a few more grinds of black pepper.

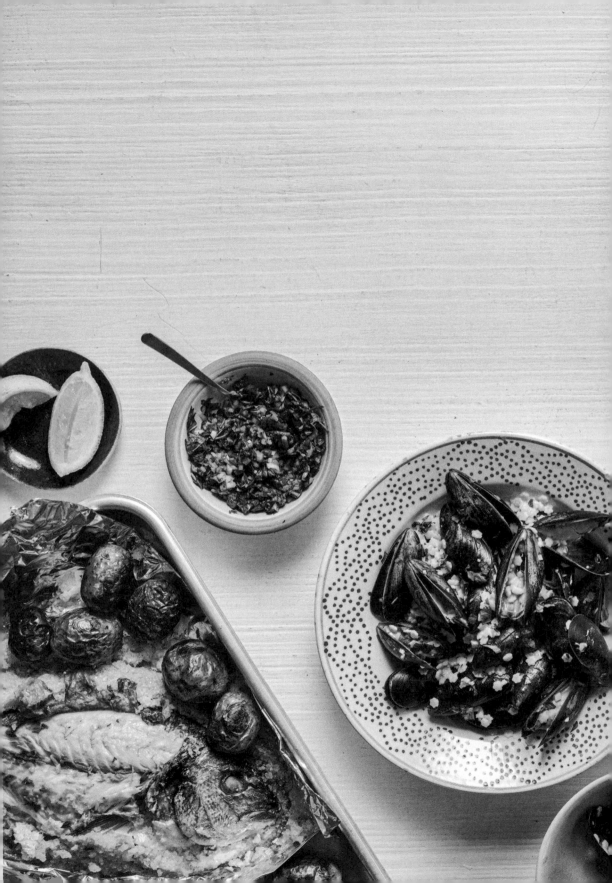

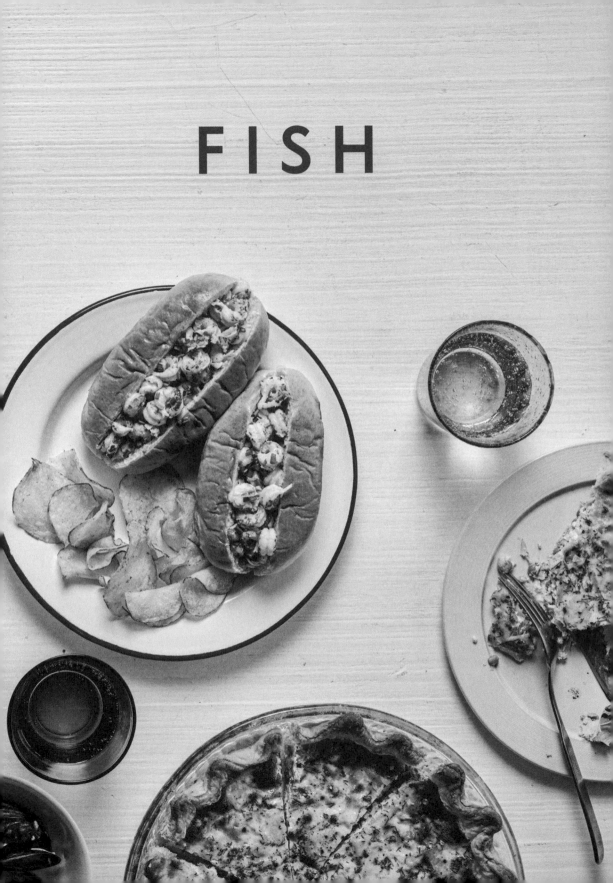

FISH

If I could describe my last meal on earth – my *Desert Island* choice, if you like – it would be early summer, warm enough to sit outside but not too hot, and I'd be sitting outside a restaurant in Cancale, France's oyster capital of Brittany, at a table overlooking the oyster beds in the harbour. To start, I'd enjoy a dozen oysters, followed by a big pot of moules marinière from La Baie de Mont Saint-Michel served with hot, crisp frites and some good French bread to dip in all of those lovely cooking juices at the bottom of the pot. I'd finish with a crêpe beurre sucre, and the whole lot would be accompanied by an unlimited supply of icy Côtes de Provence or Île de Beauté wine. For my last meal on earth I'd look to seafood to feast on, rather than a big juicy steak done over a coal fire or a perfect, aromatic, crispy-skinned and home-roasted chicken.

Hands up who cooks fish at home? Most of you? Okay then. Hands up who cooks something other than salmon fillets, something with prawns, or, at a push, a fancy, homemade version of fish and chips? Fillets of sea bass that come with those little pats of pre-flavoured butter, or a bag of defrosted mixed seafood folded into tomato pasta? If you've not put up your hand, I feel you. Most people I know would love to have more confidence when cooking fish at home, and I'm guessing that if you've picked up a copy of this book, you're looking to try something new.

I learned two important things when writing this chapter. First, that even though I love almost every single piece of fish and seafood under the sun, cooked or raw (except whelks: why the French insist on putting the horrible, bitter, rubbery things on their fruit de mer platters I don't know), I was a little bit intimidated about writing recipes that were designed to teach others to do so. Fish and seafood are expensive, there is no denying it, and the difference between overcooked and undercooked can be just moments. Second, that out of my friends who were kind enough to offer to test some of these recipes for me, no one seemed to want to go near the fish section. As a nation, why are we so intimidated by cooking fish at home?

To try and help you through the process, none of the recipes in this chapter are complicated. I know the **Whole Roast Sea Bass with Fennel and Potatoes** (page 174) and **Whole Baked Fish in a**

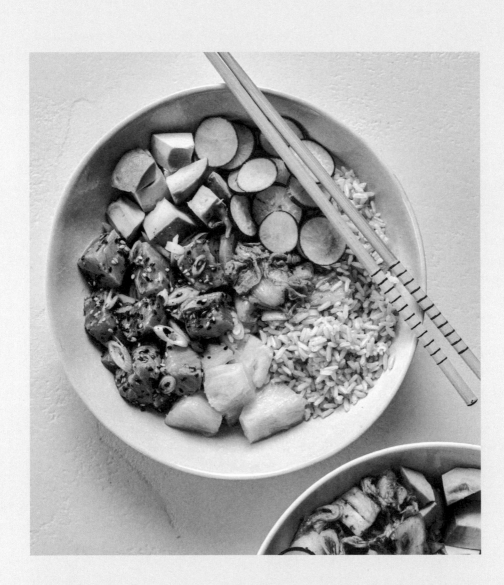

Sea Salt Crust (page 178) may sound intimidating, but really they're among the simplest in this book. I've also included recipes for **Easy Salmon Poke Bowls** on page 164, and my absolute favourite **Korean Sashimi Salad** (page 156), which are really easy jumping-off points if you're also sustaining my level of sushi and sashimi addiction, and are keen to start working with raw fish at home.

Korean Sashimi Salad (*Hwe Dup Bap*)

SERVES 2

Preparation time: 10 minutes
Cooking time: 20 minutes

For the sashimi salad
110g (½ cup) brown basmati rice
½ cucumber
2 large radishes
2 large spring onions
150g (5oz) sushi-grade salmon
150g (5oz) sushi-grade tuna
2 large handful of baby leaf
  salad leaves
1 tsp sesame seeds or furikake

For the Korean sweet chilli sauce
2 tbsp gochujang
1½ tbsp rice wine vinegar
1 tbsp runny honey
1 tsp toasted sesame oil

If you love poke, you are going to adore *hwe dup bap* – Korea's answer to a sashimi salad. This bowlful of tender raw tuna, fatty salmon and crunchy cucumber served over nutty brown rice is just delicious with the Korean sweet chilli sauce. Eating raw fish – especially raw tuna – can be dangerous if you don't take adequate care, so do check with your fishmonger that it is sushi-grade. If they are as nice as mine, they'll also remove the skin for you too – something that is tricky to do well at home unless you have a really, really sharp knife.

1. Cook the rice in a saucepan of boiling water for 20 minutes. Cook it like pasta, in a lot of water, rather than measuring everything out; using the absorption method is the easiest way to burn rice, and besides, unless you've cooked the recipe ahead you're going to be running it under the cold tap to rapidly cool it anyway!

2. To prepare your salad ingredients, peel and roughly cube the cucumber, cut the radishes into thin batons and shred the spring onions. Carefully slice the skin off your salmon if the fishmonger has not done it for you, and cube both pieces of fish into bite-sized pieces.

3. To make the sauce, whisk together the gochujang, rice wine vinegar, honey and sesame oil until smooth.

4. Once you've cooled and drained your rice, divide it between two bowls and sprinkle over the cucumber, radishes, spring onions and salad leaves. Throw the fish on top and drizzle with a generous amount of the sauce. Sprinkle with sesame seeds or furikake and serve with the bowl of sauce alongside so you can add more as you eat.

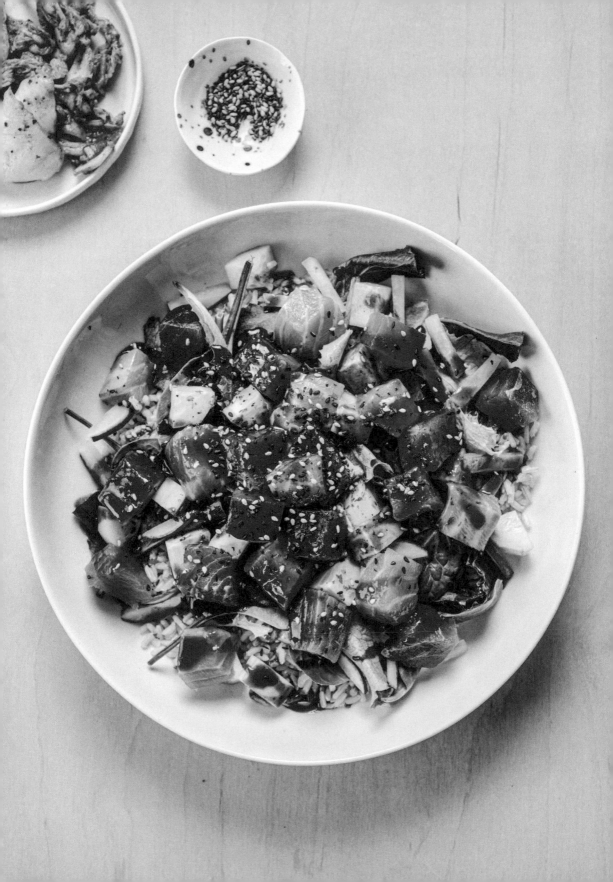

Beetroot and Dill Cured Salmon

SERVES 3–4

Preparation time: 10 minutes

70g (2½oz) raw beetroot
70g (¼ cup) rock salt
70g (⅓ cup) golden caster sugar
25ml (1½ tbsp) gin
juice of ½ lemon
small handful of fresh dill
250–300g (9–10oz) salmon tail

Curing salmon is a wonderful way to get a side of salmon to go a bit further, and looks really impressive when you serve it for guests. I tend to buy a big side, and slice and freeze a few fillets out of the thick end before curing the tail. This is a very classic cure made with beetroot to give both a bit of an earthy flavour, and a beautiful contrast between the bright orange salmon and the jewel-like beet staining around the edges. Serve it as a canapé on top of homemade blini pancakes with a dab of soured cream and a sprig of dill, or as a topping for a super-indulgent plate of avocado toast (both on page 160).

1. Roughly chop the beetroot and blitz it in a blender or food processor with the salt, sugar, gin, lemon juice and dill to make a rough paste.

2. Pat any excess moisture off the salmon with kitchen paper, then lay it, skin side down, on a double layer of clingfilm. Place the salmon on the clingfilm and then transfer to a small dish in which the salmon just fits snugly.

3. Pour the cure mixture over the salmon so that it is completely covered, folding the excess flaps of clingfiilm over the top so you've got a sealed package inside the dish. Refrigerate for 48 hours.

4. Wearing a pair of disposable gloves, gently rinse the cure off the salmon under the cold tap and pat dry with kitchen paper.

5. Lay the salmon, skin side down, on a chopping board. Using a big, flat, very sharp knife and starting at the thicker end, cut the salmon into very thin slices, slightly on the diagonal, cutting across the fillet. Don't be nervous. Think of a slice of smoked salmon, and go long and thin. You'll start with little

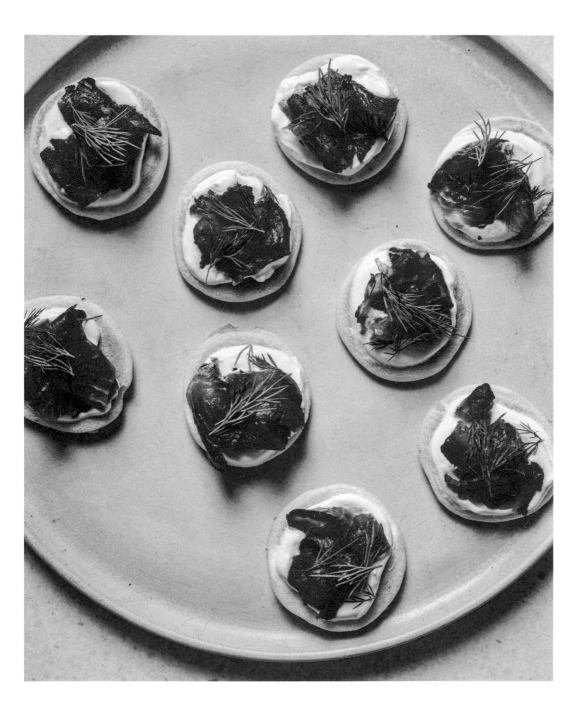

pieces at first, but practice makes perfect! Or, if you can't get the hang of it, simply run the sharp knife along the bottom of the fillet, removing the skin, and cut 5mm (¼in) slices at a 90-degree angle for a fancy gastropub-style starter.

Homemade Blini Pancakes

MAKES 36

Preparation time: 5 minutes
Cooking time: 15 minutes

1 large egg
100g (¾ cup) plain flour
150ml (⅔ cup) milk
unsalted butter, for frying
freshly ground sea salt and black
  pepper

To serve
soured cream
cured salmon (page 158)
fresh dill

1. Separate the egg. Using a balloon whisk, beat the white until it becomes light and frothy.

2. In a separate bowl, whisk together the flour, egg yolk, milk and a generous amount of seasoning.

3. Gently stir the egg white into the flour mixture.

4. Heat a non-stick frying pan over a medium heat. Once it is hot, fry the batter a few spoonfuls at a time to make perfect small, round pancakes. If you find they are sticking, add some unsalted butter, a little at a time. Continue until you have used up all the batter.

5. Top each blini with a dab of soured cream, a piece of cured salmon and a sprig of dill before serving.

Cured Salmon Avocado Toast

SERVES 1–2

Preparation time: 5 minutes

1 large ripe avocado
2 slices of farmhouse bread,
  toasted
a few slices of cured salmon
juice of roughly ¼ lemon
handful of fresh dill, chopped
freshly ground sea salt and black
  pepper

1. Peel, stone and cut the avocado into thick slices. Lay the slices over each piece of toast and press down lightly with a fork until they're slightly crushed and sticking to the toast.

2. Lightly sprinkle each slice with sea salt before topping with the cured salmon.

3. Finish each slice with a squeeze of lemon, a sprinkling of dill and a good few grinds of black pepper.

Cornish Mussels

SERVES 2

Preparation time: 10–15 minutes
(depending on your mussels)
Cooking time: 10 minutes

500g (1lb 2oz) mussels
1 large banana shallot
large knob of unsalted butter
pinch of sea salt
50ml (3 tbsp) Cornish cider
2 ½ tbsp Cornish clotted cream
2 tbsp freshly chopped dill

The area around Padstow and the Camel Estuary boasts some beautiful coastline as well as a high concentration of the UK's best seafood and seafood restaurants. We visited for our family holiday last spring, a trip almost entirely planned around where we were going to eat. I had something similar to these mussels at a little gastropub near Bodmin and, after having earlier eaten a very heavy lunch, they hit the spot nicely. Use a chilled bottle of cider so you can drink the rest with the meal, and serve with some nice sourdough bread for dunking.

1. First, clean and de-beard your mussels (see tip). This shouldn't take long if they have come from the supermarket fish counter as they are usually pretty clean. Then transfer the mussels to the bowl of clean, cold water as you go. If any mussels are cracked or broken, discard them. If any mussels are open, hold them closed for a few seconds. If they stay closed, you're good to transfer them to the bowl. If they don't, throw them away too – it is better to be safe than sorry!

2. Peel and finely chop the shallot, and heat the butter over a medium heat in a large, lidded saucepan. Add the shallot and a pinch of sea salt and fry for about 5 minutes until the shallot is softened, but not browned.

3. Add the cider to the pan, letting the alcohol bubble away for a minute or so. Drain the mussels (use a sieve to make sure you're not adding any grit to the pan) and add them to the cider mixture. Put on the lid and allow the mussels to steam open. This should only take another couple of minutes.

4. Remove the mussels from the heat and stir in the clotted cream and the dill until all of the mussels are well coated.

5. Discard any mussels that haven't opened and serve immediately in a warm bowl.

tip

To de-beard mussels, empty and clean your kitchen sink, tip in the mussels then cover with cold water. Fill a bowl with cold water and set aside. Using a clean sponge, scrub the outside of each mussel to make sure they're clean, and if there are any 'beards' (the scruffy brown things clinging to the lip), gently tug them away.

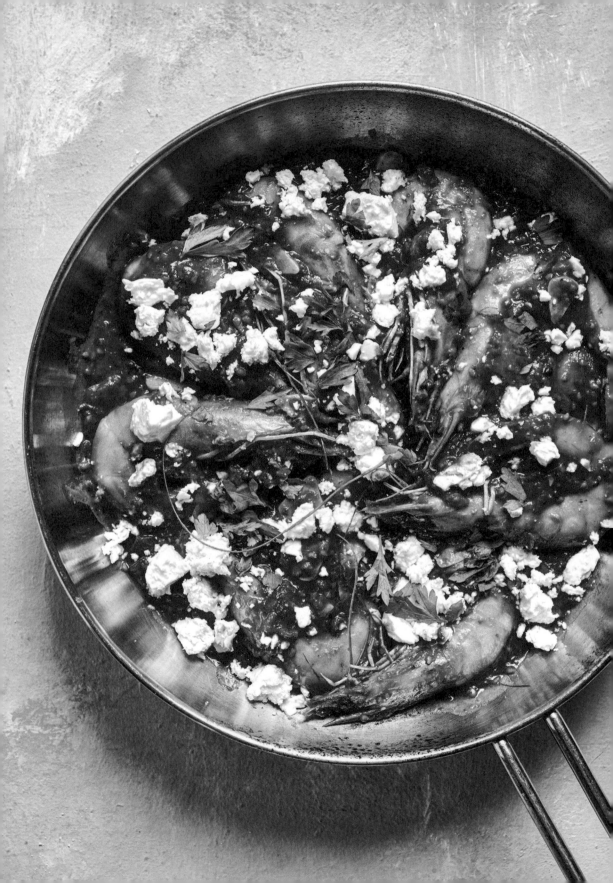

Prawn Saganaki

SERVES 2

Preparation time: 5 minutes
Cooking time: 25 minutes

3 large garlic cloves
1 tbsp extra virgin olive oil
¼ tsp Aleppo chilli flakes
100ml (6 tbsp) dry white wine
400g (14oz) tin cherry tomatoes
1 tsp golden caster sugar
¼ tsp dried oregano
8–10 raw giant king prawns
60g (2¼oz) feta
small handful of basil or flat leaf
    parsley
freshly ground sea salt and black
    pepper

I first made this Greek prawn dish after a particularly depressing afternoon flat hunting. I was starting to panic that we'd end up homeless if we couldn't find anywhere suitable, but this was an instant mood changer; by the time I reached the bottom of the bowl I was relaxed and happy again.

Chopped tomatoes will work fine here, but do make the effort to seek out whole tinned cherry tomatoes which are a total game changer. Warm ciabatta on the side to mop up the copious sauce is, for me, non-negotiable.

1. Peel and thinly slice the garlic cloves. Add them, along with the oil, to a large cold frying pan, large enough to comfortably fit all of the prawns in a single layer. Set the pan over a medium heat until the garlic has infused into the oil, and is just starting to brown. This should take 4–5 minutes.

2. Stir in the chilli flakes, followed by the white wine. Allow to bubble for another minute before adding the tomatoes, sugar, oregano and a generous amount of salt and pepper. Reduce the heat to low and allow the sauce to simmer for 15 minutes.

3. Nestle the prawns into the sauce and cook for 5 minutes, turning roughly halfway. You'll know they're done when they have just turned from grey to pink on each side.

4. Remove the pan from the heat and divide the prawns and the sauce between two warm bowls, crumbling the feta and sprinkling the basil or parsley (roughly chopped) over each one before serving.

tip

A finger bowl of warm water on the side, perhaps with a slice of fresh lemon, will be very welcome with this – things can get messy!

Easy Salmon Poke Bowls

SERVES 2

Preparation time: 15 minutes
Cooking time: 25 minutes

110g (½ cup) brown basmati rice
2 tsp dark soy sauce
1 tbsp rice wine vinegar
1 tbsp toasted sesame oil
2 tsp furikake
200g (7oz) sushi-grade salmon
1 large spring onion
large handful of fresh pineapple
1 small avocado
2 large radishes
6 tbsp kimchee

I will never say no to top-quality sushi, but for every day my favourite method of preparation is in a Hawaiian-style poke bowl, loaded up with not just cubes of oily fresh salmon tossed in a Japanese-inspired dressing, but a little bit of all my favourite colourful toppings. Mango works really well in the place of pineapple, as would some Korean cucumber pickles (page 115) in lieu of the kimchee, which I make when I've not been to Chinatown or the health food store recently. Always talk to your fishmonger about the fish you're buying to make sure it is sushi-grade and safe to eat raw, and be sure to enjoy it the same day!

1. Cook the rice in a saucepan of boiling water for 25 minutes until just tender. Unless I'm making pilau rice to serve with a curry, I never measure my water and cook my rice like pasta – I find using the traditional absorption method is the easiest way to end up with burned rice!

2. While the rice is cooking prepare the rest of your ingredients. To make the dressing for the salmon poke whisk together the soy sauce, rice vinegar, toasted sesame oil and furikake.

3. Cut the salmon into bite-sized cubes, trimming off any skin or excess fatty bits as you go. Toss the salmon in the prepared dressing.

4. Thinly slice the spring onion and cut the pineapple and avocado into bite-sized chunks. Thinly slice the radishes.

5. Once the rice is cooked, rinse it under a cold tap until cooled and drain well. (If I have time I like to cook the rice a bit in advance so I can let it cool a little at room temperature. Don't leave it for too long, though, as harmful bacteria can grow in room-temperature rice.)

6. Spoon the salmon over the rice and arrange the rest of the ingredients on top to build your ideal bowl.

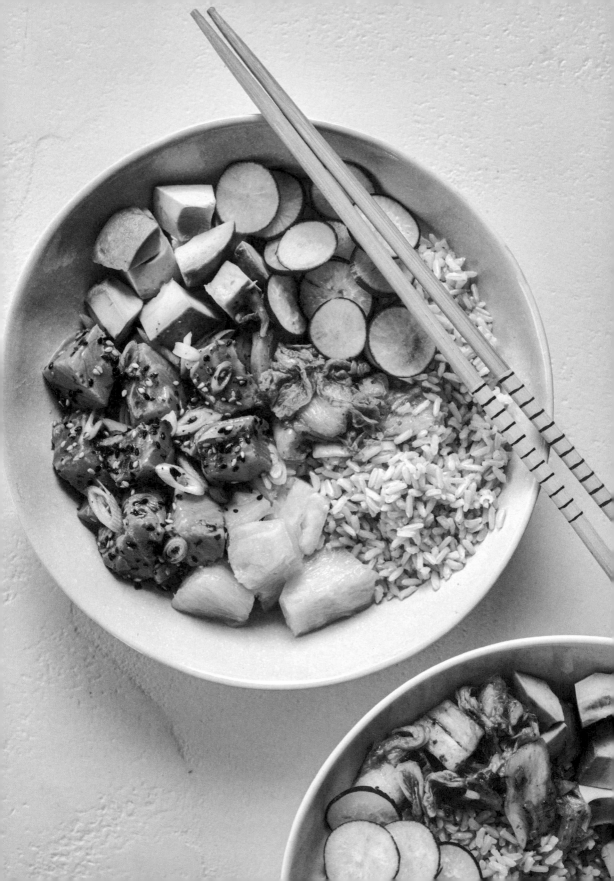

Hot Prawns in Garlic Butter

SERVES 2

Preparation time: 5 minutes
Cooking time: 10 minutes

2 large garlic cloves
55g (4 tbsp) unsalted butter
300g (10oz) cooked shell-on
   prawns
small handful of fresh flat leaf
   parsley
generous pinch of sea salt

I've got my dad to thank for this incredible way to make a lovely hot bowl of shell-on prawns in garlic butter, perfect to enjoy outside in the sunshine with a glass of wine and a French baguette. I know the amount of butter here might be intimidating but, after all, these prawns are supposed to be a treat, something to be savoured and enjoyed, and I think that – in moderation – eating something that makes you happy is just as good for you as eating something that supposedly contains a whole load of health benefits

1.   Peel and finely chop the garlic.

2.   Heat 40g (3 tbsp) of the butter in a large frying pan over a medium-low heat until the butter has melted and has started to froth. Add the garlic and cook gently for 3–4 minutes until the flavours are infused but the garlic has not yet started to brown.

3.   Add the prawns to the pan and toss so they are well coated in the garlic butter. Cook for a further 3 minutes, tossing occasionally, until the prawns are warmed through and the butter has started to get under their shells.

4.   Add the remaining butter to the pan and allow to melt. Roughly chop the parsley and stir it into the prawns along with a generous pinch of sea salt before dividing between two warm bowls (I know I always talk about serving things in warm bowls but here I really mean it – if you serve it in cold bowls the garlic butter will start to congeal and not be very nice around about halfway through eating!)

tip

The garlic butter left in the pan infused with the flavour from the prawn shells is always delicious mopped up with a piece of bread.

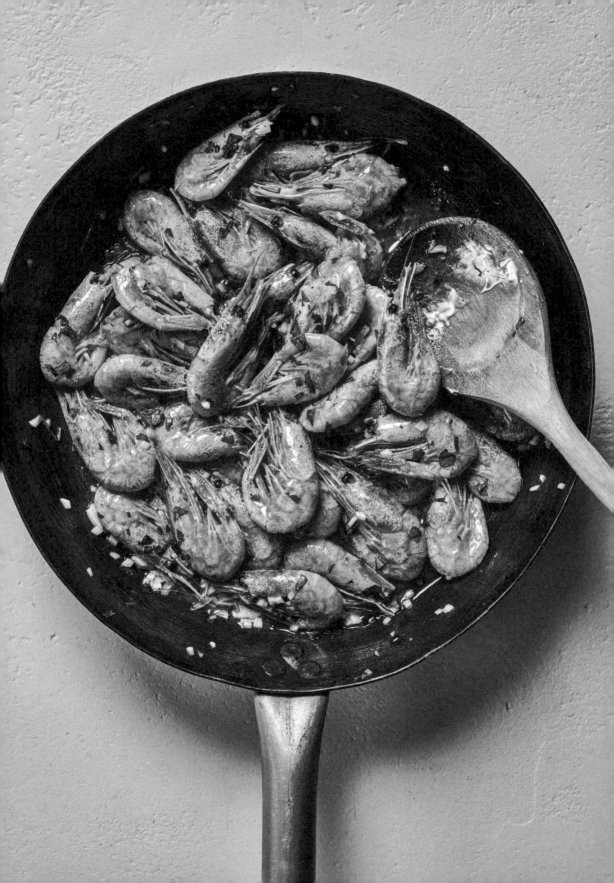

the french house ───────────

Many of my recipes are rooted in a certain time or place, either because the flavours remind me of something, somewhere or someone, or because they just happen to be what I was eating at a particular point in my life, and recalling the recipe also makes that memory instantly retrievable.

One horribly wet and rainy half-term holiday when I was about fourteen, my parents saw an advert for a traditional stone barn for sale in Brittany, northern France. Before long we were in France, looking at a sorry selection of old, run-down properties in the pouring rain.

My grandparents had recently sold the home in which I spent my summers in the Pyrenees on the French–Spanish border, so my parents thought it might be nice to have our own French holiday home, and that we should make it a bit of a conversion project.

During the trip I was instantly charmed by the sheer volume of crêpes and galettes – the savoury buckwheat filled pancakes that are the regional speciality – that Brittany had to offer. However, as well as always being cold and wet, I didn't have that magical ability my parents have to look at a ruin and imagine how it could be converted into a beautiful home. Nowhere had the internet and everywhere we looked at was pretty grim. My parents fell in love with what would later come to be our home, and soon they were arranging to buy the run-down barn (complete with straw and animal droppings on

the floor) and attached house, which, if it were possible, was in an even sorrier state.

I think it was the food in Brittany that helped me fall totally, head over heels in love with that house. Within a few years my parents had transformed it into a comfortable home full of gorgeous exposed local stone and wooden beams, a home where it was cosy to curl up in front of the fire in winter, and lovely to sit on the front patio in summer. The French House also held the first kitchen where I was the primary cook.

Ever since I was little I've had a passionate love for French supermarkets. Aside from sitting by the pool in the summer sunshine with her every afternoon, one of the strongest memories I have of spending time with my late grandmother in France were our trips to the big supermarket in Argelès. I have no idea why we needed to go as her Jewish Ma-ma genes were strong; her wall-to-wall, floor-to-ceiling pantry cupboards were always full to bursting, and there were occasions where the fridge doors had to be held shut by my father and my grandfather with bungee straps! My first food memory created in our new French house was of the local sea salt, which we discovered via the medium of my beloved supermarket. Just after some regular sea salt to cook with, my mum picked a cheap tub of Breton *fleur de sel* off the supermarket shelf. *Fleur de sel* is a wonderful salt. For a flaky sea salt it is quite fine and has small crystals that give the effect of being slightly damp in the tub, even if the salt is bone dry. It has a very mild, almost sweet flavour

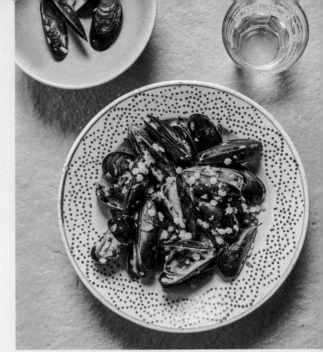

It was the local seafood that really opened up my culinary horizons and made me keen to cook shellfish at home.

– as I mentioned in my list of essential and unusual ingredients (page 14). We first enjoyed it rubbed onto the creamy pale flesh of halved home-grown courgettes – a mix of what we'd brought from home and what we were handed by our French neighbour, grown right over the garden fence – which were griddled until golden and soft on the barbecue.

While my parents' monthly trips were all about the conversion, when I came with them – first during the school holidays and later during time off from my studies and in the weeks I took off work – our first order of business was to explore. The best part of these forays was that they always came with lunch, either in the form of a pot of moules, a Breton galette or a traditional *plat du jour*. I've already mentioned the crêpes and the galettes, but it was the local seafood that really opened up my culinary horizons and made me keen to cook shellfish at home. The **Garlicky Moules with Tiny Pasta** (page 189) are testament to the many, many pots of local Normandy mussels I've put away during visits to seaside towns over the years. They're basically the Breton equivalent to our fish and chips – and I think my now well developed and

lifelong passion for Cancale oysters has helped frame my constant need to know the source of what I am eating.

Certain recipes stay rooted in a time and place because life is always changing. The taxes in France rose and my parents moved somewhere new in Kent, which changed their lifestyle, so we took the painful decision to let the house go. So many of the recipes in this book have their roots on our Brittany patio, either because I created them there, or they were inspired by something we ate on our very last visit, or because they are simply family favourites we only seemed to make in that kitchen. These recipes, such as my **Tomato, Black Olive and Courgette Bread with Anchovy Butter** overleaf, **Tomato Salad with Pomegranate Molasses** (page 121), and **Hot Prawns in Garlic Butter** (page 166) are not just recipes for me – they're memories. Memories that I will cherish forever through food, even though the time and the place they came from are now gone.

Tomato, Black Olive and Courgette Bread with Anchovy Butter

SERVES 4-6

Preparation time: 15 minutes
Cooking time: 40 minutes

100g (1 cup) grated courgette
½ tsp sea salt
100g (¾ cup) plain flour
50g (scant ½ cup) wholemeal flour
½ tsp baking powder
½ tsp bicarbonate of soda
1 large egg
75ml (⅓ cup) light olive oil
65g (⅓ cup) 0% fat Greek yogurt
25g (2 tbsp) pitted black olives
60g (1 cup) sun-dried tomatoes in oil

For the anchovy butter
55g (4 tbsp) unsalted butter
5 anchovies, packed in oil

The summer I wrote this book savoury cake-breads were everywhere in France. While we were packing up the house we stopped for lunch under a beautiful wisteria covered terrace in the local town. It was one of those funny old French places with an over-the-top menu and nineties presentation; before our *plat du jour* arrived we were served a few little vegetable bread puffs as nibbles, more like savoury cake than anything else. Then, a few days later I was reading *Saveurs*, my favourite French food magazine, when I came across not one, but two different recipes for them.

My version of this savoury cake-bread relies on sun-dried tomatoes and black olives to add a bit of a kick, as well as freshly grated courgettes from my parents' garden for some backbone. Make sure it is totally cool before you slice it; the flavour transforms when it does, so don't be tempted to eat it warm!

1. Preheat the oven to 180°C/350°F/Gas 4 and line a 450g/1lb (the smaller of the two standard sizes) loaf tin with baking parchment.

2. Toss the grated courgette with ¼ teaspoon sea salt in a small bowl and set aside.

3. In a large bowl, combine the rest of the sea salt, the flours, baking powder and bicarbonate of soda. Set aside.

4. In another small bowl, combine the egg, oil and yogurt.

5. Quarter the olives and roughly chop the sun-dried tomatoes before adding them to the dry mixture. Squeeze any excess

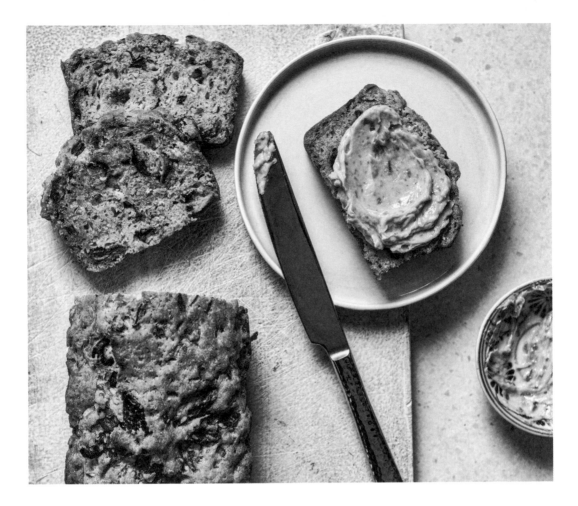

water out of the grated courgette over the kitchen sink and add that to the dry mixture as well. Fold the vegetables into the flour mix until everything is well coated.

6. Add the wet mixture to the dry and fold again until everything is combined. Transfer to the prepared loaf tin and bake in the oven for 30–40 minutes until the top is cracked and a cake tester or sharp knife inserted into the middle of the loaf comes out clean.

7. Once the tin is cool enough to touch, transfer the loaf to a wire rack to cool completely.

8. While the bread is cooling, make the anchovy butter by blending the butter and the anchovies together in a mini chopper or food processor until the mixture is smooth.

tip

This recipe makes more anchovy butter than you'll need. I love it slathered on hot toast and on my soldiers to go with a boiled egg, but to make this dish truly vegetarian good-quality salted butter would also be delicious.

Ultimate Tuna Pasta

SERVES 2

Preparation time: 5 minutes
Cooking time: 20 minutes

200g (7oz) dried pasta shapes
1 banana shallot
2 tbsp non-pareille capers
2 × 160g (5oz) tins tuna in spring
   water, drained
zest of 1 lemon
2 tbsp extra virgin olive oil
1 handful of roughly chopped
   fresh flat leaf parsley
freshly ground sea salt and black
   pepper
juice from roughly ½ lemon,
   to taste

Non-pareille capers are among my top ingredients – you can always find a jar in my fridge as I think they're perfect for adding a little hit of salt, acid and general briny astringency to whatever they come into contact with. I think banana shallots, too, are excellent; they're so mild they lend themselves well to being folded into no-cook sauces like this one.

1. Cook the pasta in a saucepan of boiling salted water as per the packet instructions.

2. Meanwhile, finely chop the shallot and the capers. Combine together with the tuna and the lemon zest, olive oil and parsley in a small bowl. Season to taste with salt, pepper and a squeeze of fresh lemon juice.

3. Drain the pasta well and return to the pan. Add the sauce and stir well until everything is combined.

tip

Non-pareille capers are baby capers and have a more delicate flavour and a much better texture than ordinary varieties. You can find them in most supermarkets and they're often better value than regular ones!

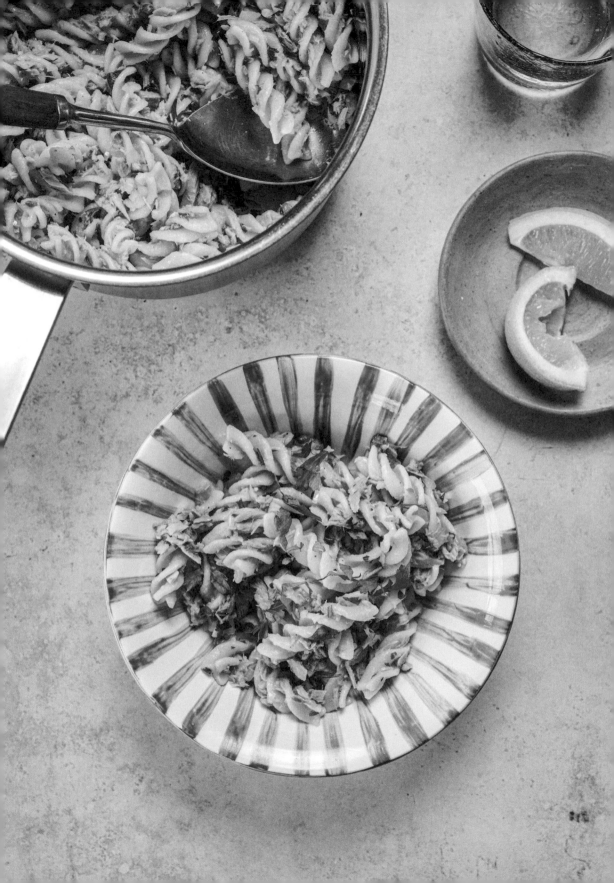

Whole Roast Sea Bass with Fennel and Potatoes

SERVES 2

Preparation time: 15 minutes
Cooking time: 1 hour

This is a special, deceptively simple, Friday night supper for two, to be shared at the table, preferably with the rest of the bottle of wine you used to braise the fennel and the potatoes.

400g (14oz) waxy potatoes
1 small fennel bulb
2 banana shallots
1 tbsp extra virgin olive oil, plus extra for drizzling
200ml (¾ cup) dry white wine
1 small sustainable whole sea bass, gutted and scaled
½ lemon
small bunch of fresh dill
freshly ground sea salt and black pepper

1. Preheat the oven to 200°C/400°F/Gas 6.

2. Peel and very thinly slice the potatoes, fennel and shallots. I do all of this on the medium setting of a mandolin so use that if you've got one, otherwise use a sharp knife.

3. Toss the sliced potatoes, fennel and shallots together with the olive oil and a generous amount of salt and pepper in a baking dish, arranging them so that they create a bed for the fish. Pour over the white wine and cover the whole thing in foil. Bake in the oven for 25 minutes.

4. Meanwhile, rinse the fish under the cold tap to make sure there's no blood left in the cavity from where it was gutted, or any stray scales still stuck to the outside. Lay the bass down on a clean chopping board and pat dry with kitchen paper.

5. Thinly slice the lemon and then stuff the slices, along with the dill, into the fish cavity. Season the cavity with more salt and pepper. If you wish, using a sharp knife, score a couple of parallel lines in the top of the fish skin.

6. Remove the foil from the fennel and potato mixture, and return to the oven for a further 15 minutes.

7. Lay the fish down on top of the potatoes. Drizzle with a little extra olive oil and return to the oven for 15–20 minutes, depending on the size of your sea bass, until you can see the flesh is white where you have scored the skin and it gently flakes when you test it with a fork.

tip

I suggest getting your sea bass from a fishmonger or a fish counter where you can ask them to gut it and descale it for you, just ask them for enough to serve two.

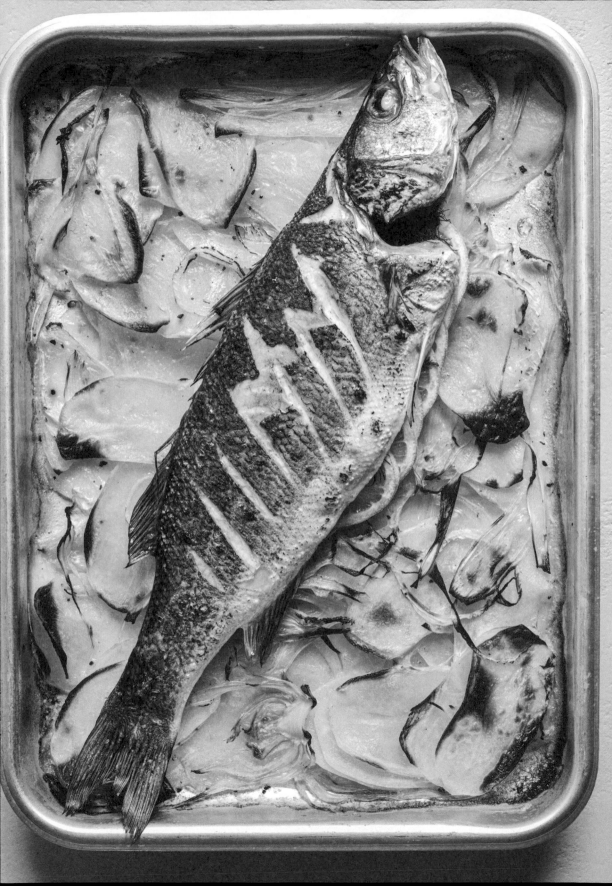

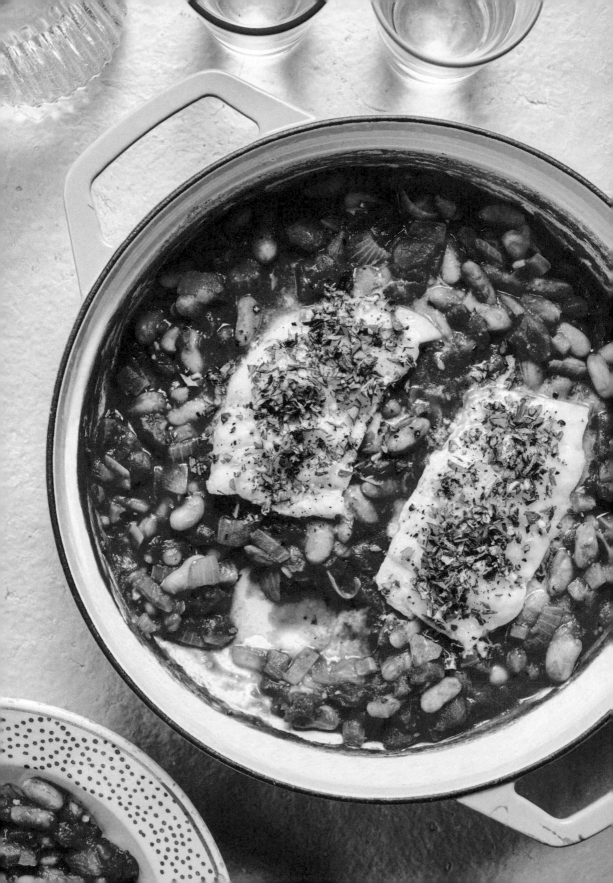

Tomato Braised Bean and White Fish Stew with Gremolata

SERVES 2

Preparation time: 10 minutes
Cooking time: 35 minutes

1 small onion
1 celery stick
1 tbsp extra virgin olive oil
1 large garlic clove
75ml (5 tbsp) dry white wine
400g (14oz) tin cannellini beans
400g (14oz) tin chopped
   tomatoes
150ml (⅔ cup) fresh fish stock
2 chunky sustainable cod fillets
freshly ground sea salt and black
   pepper

For the gremolata
1 large garlic clove
small handful of flat leaf parsley
zest of ½ lemon
small pinch of sea salt

tip

As with any sort of tomato-based fish stew, you can't go wrong serving this with a crusty loaf to mop up all the juices.

This is a lovely fresh stew that I make with cod but is nice with any chunky piece of white, sustainable fish you have available. I didn't have any white wine on hand when I first made this so, with a nod to Nigella, I made it with white vermouth instead. It added a really unusual element to the tomato stew that I quite liked, but found rather polarising, so afterwards I reverted to using dry white wine. Try it if you want to enhance the sweetness of the tomatoes and the fish stock.

1. Peel and finely chop the onion and the celery stick.

2. Heat the olive oil in a large, lidded shallow casserole dish over a medium heat and gently fry the onions and the celery for about 10 minutes until they are soft, but not browned. Peel and finely chop the garlic and add it to the pan, gently frying for a further minute until aromatic.

3. Add the white wine to the pan and allow it to bubble gently while you drain the beans and add them to the pan with a generous amount of salt and pepper. Then add the tinned tomatoes, followed by the stock. Turn the heat up to high until it is bubbling, then reduce it to low to simmer, uncovered, for 10 minutes.

4. Make the gremolata by peeling and finely chopping the garlic, finely chopping the parsley and mixing them together in a small bowl along with the lemon zest and sea salt. Set aside.

5. Nestle the two fish fillets between the beans and season the tops with salt and pepper. Place the lid on the pan and allow the fish to steam for 10 minutes until the fish is cooked through and you can flake it gently with a fork.

6. Serve the bean stew in two warm bowls, each topped with a fish fillet, and the gremolata piled on top of the fish.

Whole Baked Fish
in a Sea Salt Crust

SERVES 2
Preparation time: 15 minutes
Cooking time: 50 minutes

300g (10oz) baby Jersey royal
    potatoes
glug of light oil
360g (1⅓ cups) coarse sea salt
1 large egg white
1 small sustainable sea bass or
    sea bream, gutted and scaled

For the salsa verde
1 small banana shallot
1 tbsp red wine vinegar
25g (1 cup) fresh flat leaf parsley
1 tbsp non-pareille capers
2 anchovies, packed in oil
2 tbsp extra virgin olive oil
sea salt

tip

*I suggest getting your sea bass
from a fishmonger or a fish
counter where you can ask them
to gut it and descale it for you, just
ask them for enough to serve two.*

While serving up a whole fish seems fancy, in reality it is
the answer for a really simply yet tasty supper. This recipe
for a whole baked fish – I use bass or bream, whatever is
cheap on the fish counter that day – involves three steps:
baking it in a salt and egg white crust, tossing some whole
new potatoes in a roasting tin, and a bit of chopping to
make an easy salsa verde to spoon over everything. It's so
satisfying to crack the salt crust with the side of your fork
to reveal the fish underneath.

1. Preheat the oven to 250°C/500°F/Gas 9. Finely chop the
    shallot and mix with the red wine vinegar in a bowl. Set aside.

2. Toss the potatoes, whole, together with a generous glug of oil
    on a baking tray and bake in the oven for 25 minutes.

3. Meanwhile, combine the sea salt and the egg white into a
    thick paste. Rinse the fish under the cold tap to wash off any
    stray scales or any blood left in the cavity from being gutted,
    before patting it dry on a piece of kitchen paper. Lay the fish
    out on a piece of foil and gently press the salt over the fish,
    completely covering the fish with a thin crust.

4. Remove the tray from the oven and turn the temperature
    down to 200°C/400°F/Gas 6. Transfer the foil sheet with
    the crusted fish on to the tray next to the potatoes and return
    to the oven for a further 25 minutes. You'll be able to tell it is
    done when the crust starts to turn golden and crack.

5. Meanwhile, finish the salsa verde. Roughly chop the parsley,
    capers and anchovies and stir into the vinegar shallot mixture.
    Season to taste with a pinch of sea salt.

6. Serve the whole fish on the table between you, cracking the
    crust to reveal more of the fish as you eat.

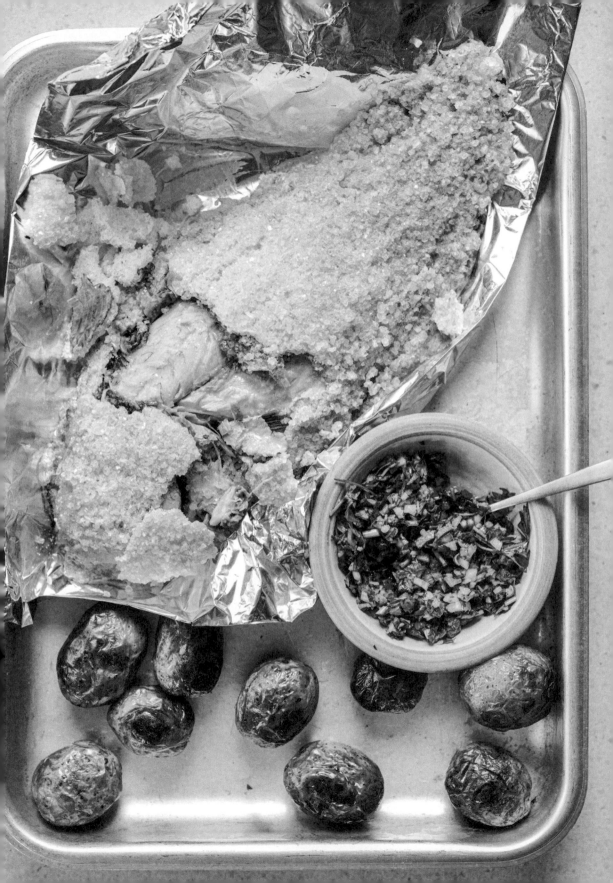

Cajun Salmon Traybake with Tropical Fruit Salsa

SERVES 2

Preparation time: 10 minutes
Cooking time: 30 minutes

1 large red pepper
1 large orange or yellow pepper
1 large red onion
2 tbsp light oil
400g (14oz) tin black beans
juice of 1 lime
2 salmon fillets
1½ tsp Cajun spice mix
1 ripe papayas
2 passion fruit
freshly ground sea salt and black
  pepper

Cajun spice mix is a total hero ingredient in my pantry – and essential to making my **Slow Cooker Mixed Bean Chilli** on page 126 – here it is simply seasoning some salmon to be baked with mixed peppers and tender black beans, some of which get slightly crispy in the oven. However, it is the tropical fruit salsa that really brings the whole dish together. I really like the flavour of papaya, but if it is not for you, feel free to use some really ripe mango instead.

1. Preheat the oven to 200°C/400°F/Gas 6. Core and deseed the peppers, peel the onions and roughly chop everything into bite-sized pieces. Toss everything with 1 tablespoon of the oil and a generous amount of salt and pepper on a large baking tray. Roast in the oven for 20 minutes.

2. Meanwhile, drain and rinse the black beans and toss them with ¼ of the lime juice. Set aside.

3. Marinate the salmon by combining the Cajun spice mix, half the remaining lime juice and the remaining oil in a small bowl before adding the salmon, rubbing the marinade into the fillets to make sure they're well coated.

4. To make the salsa, halve, deseed, peel and chop the papayas and toss in a small bowl with the seeds from the passion fruits, a good few grinds of sea salt and the remaining lime juice, to taste. Set aside.

5. Toss the peppers and onions together with the black beans on the baking tray and nestle the two salmon fillets among them, pouring any excess marinade over the top of each. Roast for a further 10 minutes until the salmon is flaky but still a little pink in the middle. Serve with the tropical fruit salsa.

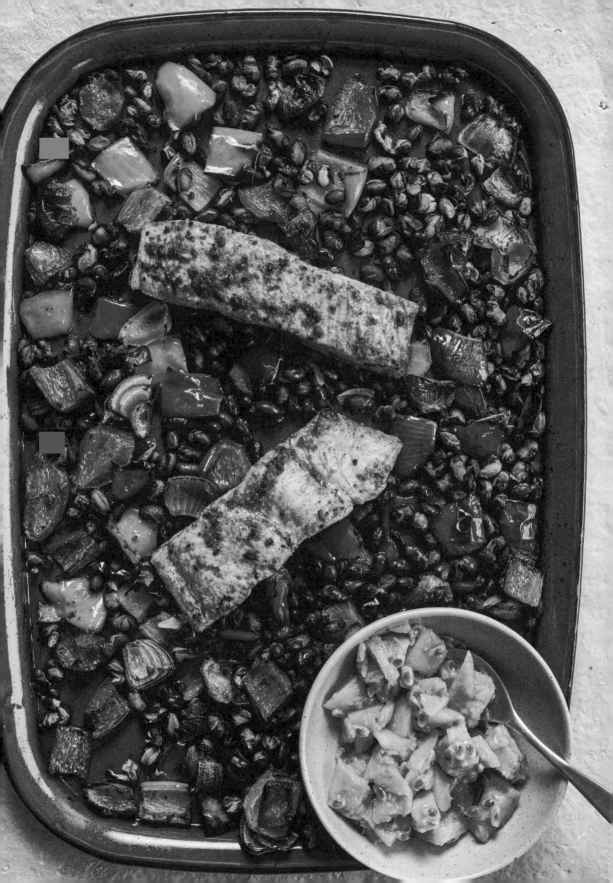

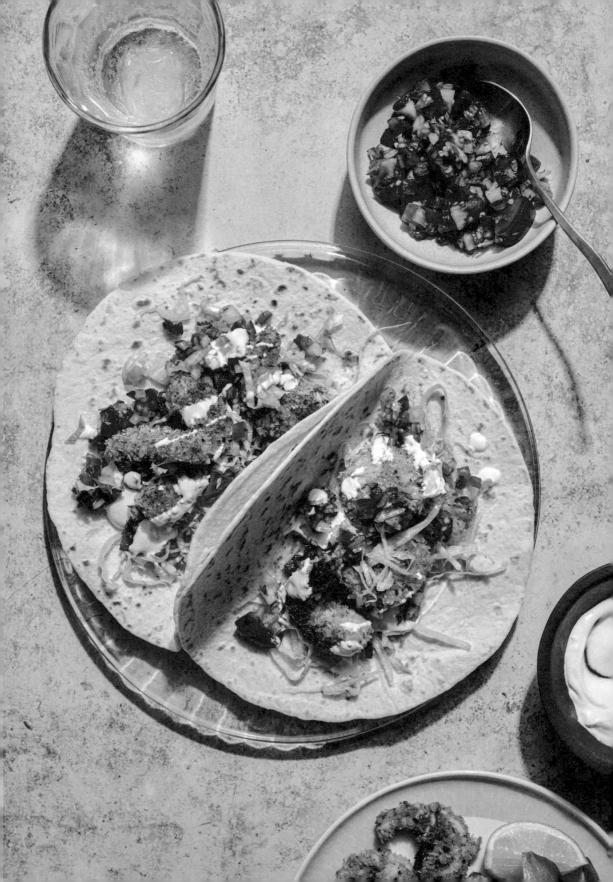

Crispy Cajun Coconut Prawn Tacos

SERVES 2

Preparation time: 10 minutes
Cooking time: 10 minutes

6 tbsp panko breadcrumbs
3 tbsp desiccated coconut
1 tbsp Cajun spice mix
3 tbsp plain flour
1 small egg
200g (7oz) raw king prawns
light oil, for frying

To serve
6–8 soft flour taco wraps
fresh salsa
shredded iceberg lettuce
soured cream

These speedy weeknight tacos contain all my favourite flavours – juicy, coconut-coated prawns, a bright, punchy fresh salsa, crunchy lettuce and cooling soured cream. These make for a pretty light meal, so perhaps serve them alongside the **Mexican Roasted Sweet Potato Salad** on page 28, the **Watermelon, Avocado and Feta Salad with Lime Dressing** on page 68 or the **Grilled Mexican Street Corn Salad** on page 73.

1. Combine the panko breadcrumbs, desiccated coconut and Cajun spice mix in a small bowl and set aside. Place the flour in another small bowl and the egg, lightly beaten, in another.

2. Pat off any excess liquid on the prawns with a piece of kitchen paper. To bread them, dip them first in the flour, then in the egg, and then in the breadcrumb–coconut mix, and set each aside on a spare plate until you run out of prawns. (So I don't accidentally breadcrumb my fingers I use one hand for dipping into the dry ingredients, and another for the wet!)

3 Gently heat enough oil to cover the bottom of a medium frying pan over a high heat until the oil is shimmering. Add the prawns in a single layer, working in two batches, frying for a few minutes on each side until uniformly golden. Set them on an additional plate lined with kitchen paper to soak up any excess oil between batches.

4. Serve the prawns hot with soft flour taco wraps, salsa, shredded lettuce and soured cream.

Black Olive Tapenade Cod with Summer Vegetables

SERVES 2

Preparation time: 10 minutes
Cooking time: 45 minutes

For the black olive tapenade cod

2 thick, sustainable cod fillets
1 large garlic clove
zest and juice of ½ lemon
1½ tbsp extra virgin olive oil
1–2 tbsp black olive tapenade
small handful of roughly
    chopped fresh flat leaf parsley
freshly ground sea salt and black
    pepper

For the summer vegetables

300g (10oz) new potatoes
1 large red pepper
1 large orange pepper
juice of ½ lemon
1 large garlic clove
1 tbsp extra virgin olive oil
150g (¾ cup) cherry tomatoes

This summery, colourful, one-pan cod dish is inspired by a rather more elegant one I had on holiday in the Dordogne. Served over a bed of fluffy polenta and a pile of roasted courgettes, my cod arrived with a black coat of tapenade, a jaunty sprig of rosemary sticking out the top, and a warm sauce of fresh chopped tomatoes, slivers of tender garlic and yet more chopped black olives spooned over it all. It was utterly delicious, but no one wants to go to that amount of effort on a weeknight, which is where my version comes in; switching the courgettes for hardy rainbow peppers, and the fussy polenta for lemon and garlic scented new potatoes.

1. Preheat the oven to 200°C/400°F/Gas 6. Marinate the cod by placing the fillets in a plastic bag along with the crushed garlic clove, lemon zest and juice, olive oil, and a generous amount of salt and pepper. Tie a knot in the top of the bag and massage gently to make sure the fish is well coated. Set aside.

2. Core and roughly chop the peppers into bite-sized pieces, and halve the potatoes. Toss together with the lemon juice, garlic clove – peeled and crushed – olive oil and a generous amount of salt and pepper in a large casserole dish. Transfer to the oven and roast for 15 minutes.

3. Toss the vegetables together so that they cook evenly, then add the tomatoes. Return to the oven for a further 15 minutes.

4. Remove the cod from the marinade and lay over the top of the veggies. Spoon the tapenade over the top of each fillet, gently smoothing to the edges of each to create what will become a crust once removed from the oven.

5. Bake the fish for a further 15 minutes before sprinkling with parsley. Serve still in the casserole dish.

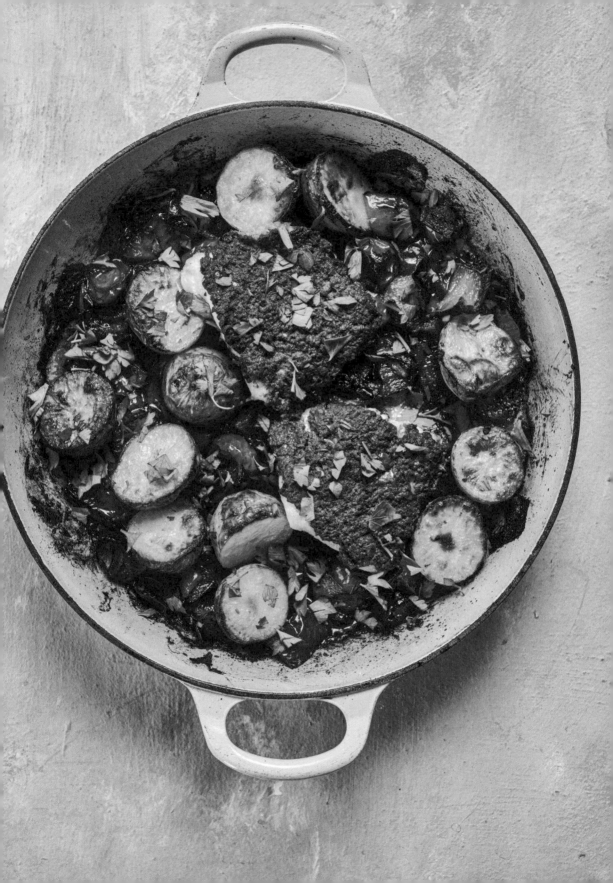

One Pan Smoked Salmon Kedgeree

SERVES 1–2

Preparation time: 5 minutes
Cooking time: 10 minutes

25g (2 tbsp) unsalted butter
2 spring onions
½ small green chilli
50g (⅓ cup) frozen petit pois
1 tsp ground turmeric
½ tsp garam masala
75g (3oz) smoked salmon
1 × 250g (9oz) pouch brown
 basmati rice
small handful of fresh coriander
2–4 eggs
freshly ground sea salt and black
 pepper

*If you've made my **Beetroot and Dill Cured Salmon** on page 158 you can use this instead of the smoked salmon.*

I've always loved the idea of kedgeree – a bowlful of curried rice at breakfast time flaked through with neon-yellow smoked haddock and crowned with a hard-boiled egg. I don't like smoked haddock but I've solved that by using smoked salmon instead, which cooks beautifully, and I've used garam masala as I can't stand regular curry powder. To make this a one pan wonder (and because everything is better with a runny yolk) I've baked the eggs in the rice just before serving. My little twist on a Victorian breakfast classic.

1. Melt the butter in a casserole dish or large, non-stick frying pan over a medium heat.

2. Top, tail and slice the spring onions and add them to the pan along with the chilli, deseeded and thinly sliced, and the petit pois. Fry everything gently for a minute or two until the chilli is soft and sizzling and the peas have defrosted and heated through.

3. Add the spices and fry for another minute or so until fragrant.

4. Slice the salmon into thin ribbons and add to the pan along with the rice and a generous amount of salt and pepper. Before you open the pouch of rice, squeeze it gently to break up the lumps.

5. Gently fry the rice mixture until the individual grains are well coated in buttery spices and the salmon has started to turn translucent.

6. Roughly chop the coriander and stir it into the rice, turning the heat down to low. Check the seasoning, then make wells in the rice to crack each egg into.

7. Cook the eggs for 3–4 minutes until the yolk is just set. I like this served with generous amounts of sriracha hot sauce.

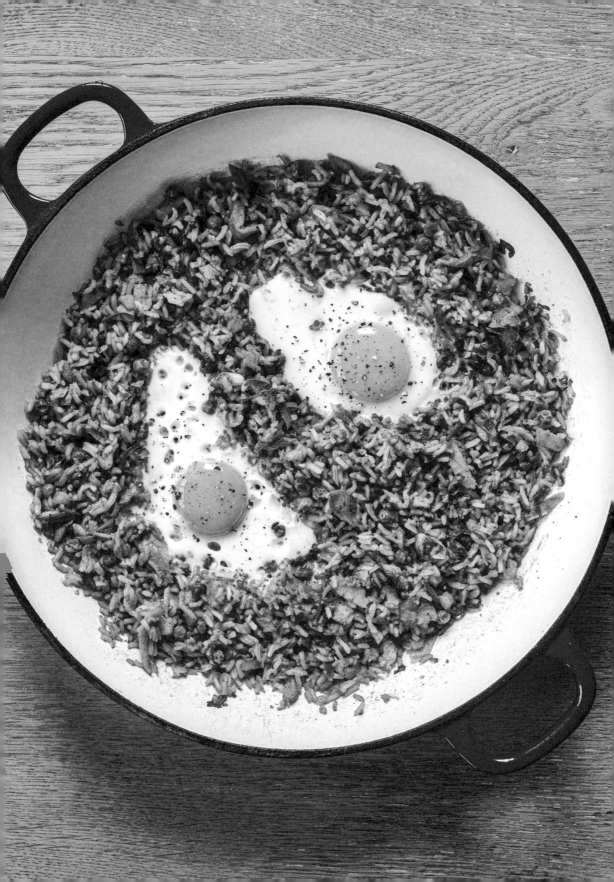

Pasta Shells with Fresh Tomato, Crab and Basil

SERVES 1

Preparation time: 5 minutes
Cooking time: 20 minutes

100g (3½oz) pasta shells
70g (3oz) mixed colour cherry
    tomatoes
small handful of fresh basil
100g (3½oz) dressed crab
1 tsp extra virgin olive oil
freshly ground sea salt and black
    pepper
juice of roughly ¼ lemon

This simple pasta dish is a celebration of summer. Juicy tomatoes, bright green torn basil, and rich dressed crab, all tossed together with pasta shells that capture the crab meat with their gentle ridges and voluptuous curves. I've made this a single serving as an indulgent treat but feel free to scale it up for an extra-special date night dish. You need only 100g (3½oz) of crab meat here whether you buy a whole dressed crab, or just the meat.

1. Cook the pasta in a saucepan of boiling salted water as per the packet instructions – as always, check it after around 10 minutes.

2. Roughly chop the tomatoes and the basil.

3. Drain the pasta and return it to the pan along with the chopped tomatoes and basil, dressed crab and olive oil. Stir gently until everything is combined, and season to taste with salt, pepper and a squeeze of fresh lemon juice.

Garlicky Moules with Tiny Pasta

SERVES 2

Preparation time: 15 minutes
Cooking time: 15 minutes

500g (1lb 2oz) mussels
30g (2 tbsp) unsalted butter
4 very large garlic cloves
120ml (½ cup) white wine
90g (3½oz) tiny pasta shapes
2 tbsp crème fraîche
large handful of fresh curly or
    flat leaf parsley
freshly ground sea salt and black
pepper

This is a very different beast to the **Cornish Mussels** on page 161. I made this for dinner one night sitting out on the patio in front of our French house with local Normandy mussels, white wine from the Loire and lots of good Brittany butter. It's the tiny pasta shapes that make this dish special, soaking up the broth and getting trapped in the mussel shells. You don't need a fork to eat this, just scoop them with the mussel shells along with the plump orange middles. Buy the smallest pieces of pasta you can find – the ones designed to cook really quickly in soups and stews.

1. First prepare the mussels (page 161).

2. Heat the butter in a medium, lidded saucepan over a medium heat until it is frothy. Peel and finely chop the garlic and gently fry in the butter for 2–3 minutes until soft and aromatic, but not at all brown.

3. Add the wine to the pan along with a generous amount of salt and pepper and stir in the pasta. If the pasta is not completely covered in the liquid, add a little more wine or a splash of water. Allow to bubble away for 5 minutes or so until the pasta is just tender.

4. Add the mussels to the pan and shake well to make sure they're well coated with the wine and pasta mixture. Put on the lid and allow the shells to steam for 5 minutes or so until the shells have opened and the pasta is tender.

5. Discard any unopened shells and stir in the crème fraîche. Transfer the mussels and pasta to a couple of big, warm bowls (with another empty one on the side for discarded shells), and finish by sprinkling the chopped parsley on top.

Spinach and Oatmeal Pancakes

SERVES 2

Preparation time: 20 minutes
Cooking time: 10 minutes

1 large egg
140ml (½ cup) buttermilk
¼ tsp bicarbonate of soda
4 tbsp plain flour
4 tbsp porridge oats
25g (½ cup) fresh spinach
light oil, for frying
freshly ground sea salt and black
   pepper

To serve
crème fraîche
½ tsp chopped chives
1 ripe avocado
smoked salmon

I love the way green pancakes look when they're in a tower. I started out by making matcha pancakes with a raspberry coulis for a Pancake Day blog post – and before I knew it I was blitzing up my pancake batter with fresh spinach leaves to try and get a healthy green hue. I'd happily enjoy these pancakes at any time of day, but I think they're best served for weekend brunch.

1. Combine the egg, buttermilk, bicarbonate of soda, flour, oats, spinach and a generous amount of salt and pepper in a high-speed blender or food processor. Blitz until you have a smooth batter.

2. Heat a generous splash of oil in a large, non-stick frying pan. Working in batches, fry the pancakes for a few minutes on each side until just golden. Keep a warm plate to hand on which to rest the cooked pancakes.

3. Top the pancakes with dollops of crème fraîche, a sprinkle of chives and another few grinds of black pepper. Serve with sliced avocado and torn smoked salmon.

tip

To get ahead, measure out all the pancake ingredients the night before into the body of your blender, just leaving out the bicarbonate of soda to add later, and leave it in the fridge so you're ready to go.

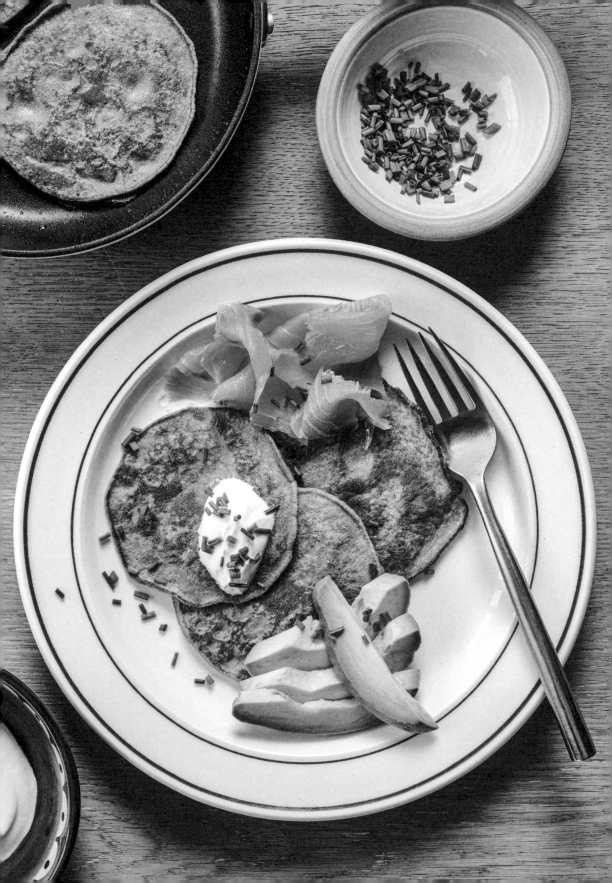

Smoked Salmon Spaghetti

SERVES 2

Preparation time: 5 minutes
Cooking time: 20 minutes

200g (7oz) spaghetti
60g (2¼oz) smoked salmon
zest of 1 lemon
2 tbsp finely snipped fresh chives
4 tbsp double cream
freshly ground sea salt and black
  pepper

I handwrite all my recipes in a kitchen notebook using different coloured biros so that I can see where and when I have made changes and revisions. I made this simple recipe for smoked salmon spaghetti as the result of a fridge raid one lunchtime. I seem to have nailed it first time as the whole thing is written in red pen. I scribbled a single word in the top right hand corner of the page, which I think pretty much sums up the dish: luscious.

1. Cook the spaghetti as per the packet instructions in a saucepan of boiling salted water; this can take anything from 10–15 minutes so do test as you go.

2. Meanwhile, slice the salmon into thin slivers and prepare the lemon zest and the chives.

3. Drain the pasta well and return it to the pan, setting it over a low, gentle heat.

4. Add the salmon, lemon zest, chives and cream to the spaghetti and stir well to combine. Season to taste with salt and pepper – be careful here, smoked salmon can be quite salty in itself – and serve immediately.

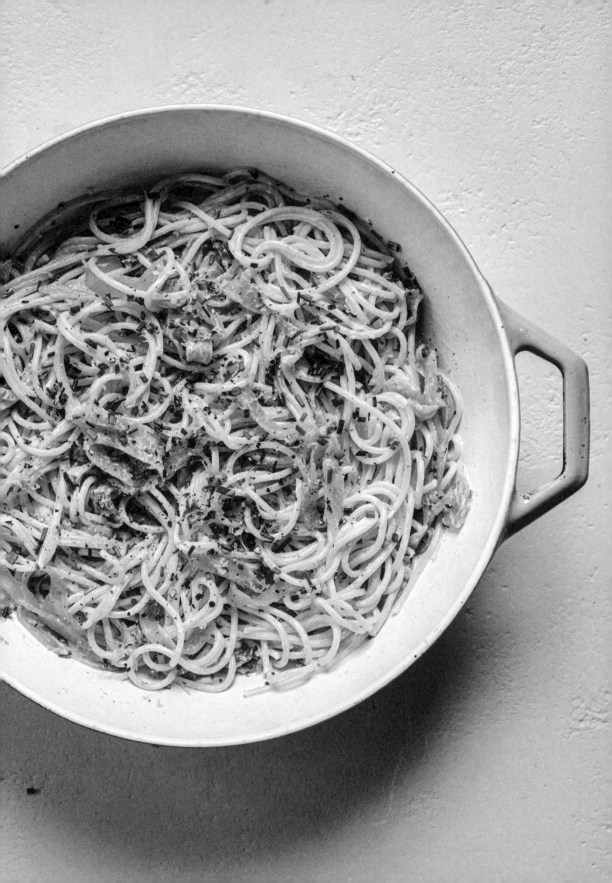

Classic Crayfish Rolls

SERVES 4

Preparation time: 10 minutes
Cooking time: 10 minutes

4 brioche hot dog rolls
unsalted butter, at room
   temperature
280g (9½oz) crayfish tails
4 tsp light mayonnaise
juice of roughly ½ lemon
small handful of fresh chives
freshly ground sea salt and black
   pepper

These crayfish rolls are my response to a wonderful lobster roll I had at a restaurant called Son of a Gun in Los Angeles. Lobster, although native to the UK, is rather pricey, so I've replaced it with crayfish instead, which you can buy tubs of in the supermarket. If you can't find any, cooked king prawns would also make a good substitute.

1. Pull apart the brioche rolls and generously butter the exposed tears on each side.

2. Heat a non-stick frying pan over a medium-high heat. Toast the buttered sections of each roll until golden, and set aside.

3. Meanwhile, combine the crayfish tails with the mayonnaise, lemon juice and a generous amount of salt and pepper, to taste.

4. Split the rolls down the middle and divide the dressed crayfish between each one. Snip a couple of chives over the exposed strip of crayfish on each one before serving.

tip

Serve these rolls either with a green salad or American-style with a handful of ready salted crisps on the side.

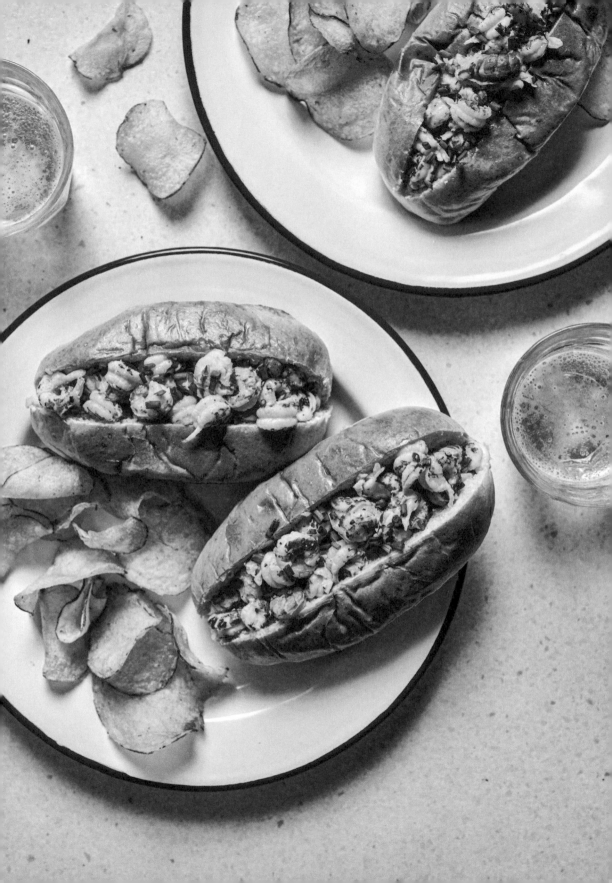

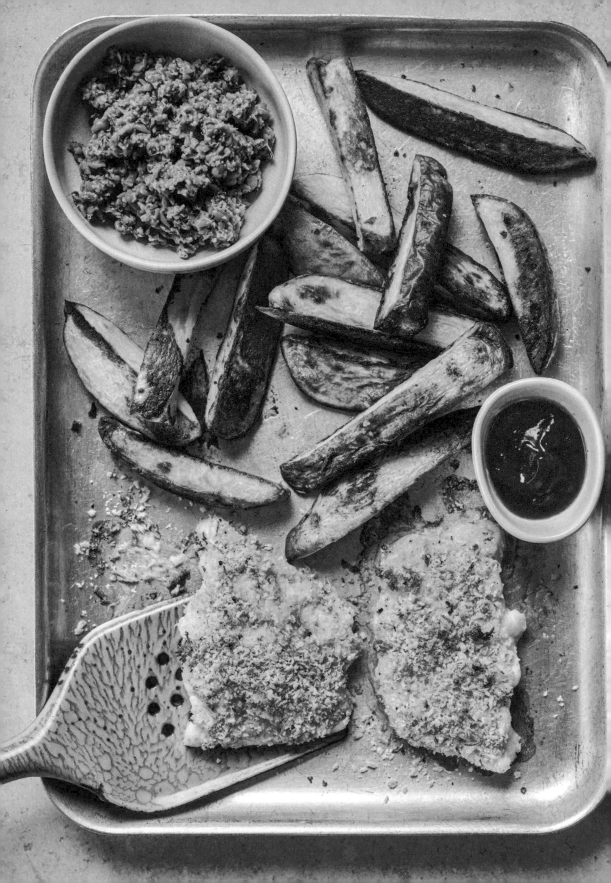

Fancy Friday Night Fish and Chips

SERVES 2

Preparation time: 10 minutes
Cooking time: 30 minutes

500g (1lb 2oz) potatoes
½ tbsp light oil
2 large pieces of sustainable
  white cod
1 tsp light mayonnaise
2 tbsp panko breadcrumbs
zest of ½ lemon
freshly ground sea salt and black
  pepper

For the mushy peas
100g (⅔ cup) frozen petit pois,
  defrosted
zest of ½ lemon
small handful of fresh mint
1 tsp extra virgin olive oil

I used to work in an office on the seafront which, naturally, was lined with fish and chip shops. While I did sometimes treat myself to a bag of chips, I've always found chip shop fish way too fatty to enjoy properly. This is where the idea for this one-tray fish and chip supper came from; proper, chunky, skin-on chips, served with baked breadcrumb-topped cod, and a fresh, vibrant side of mushy peas. Serve with a generous amount of malt vinegar, which is essential to any truly British fish supper.

1. Preheat the oven to 220°C/425°F/Gas 7. Cut the potatoes into chunky chips and toss together with the light oil and a pinch of sea salt. Bake for 20 minutes until golden.

2. Meanwhile, spread a very thin layer of mayonnaise across the top of each fish fillet. Mix together the panko breadcrumbs, lemon zest, some salt and pepper and sprinkle over the fish.

3. Toss the chips on the pan so they cook evenly. Reduce the oven temperature to 200°C/400°F/Gas 6, then nestle the breaded fish fillets among the chips, and bake for a further 10 minutes until the fish has just cooked through and the breadcrumbs are golden.

4. While the fish is cooking, make the mushy peas by blending all the ingredients together in a small food processor. Serve alongside the fish and chips.

Fried Whitebait Sandwich

SERVES 2

Preparation time: 5 minutes
Cooking time: 5 minutes

200g (7oz) frozen whitebait,
  defrosted
2 tbsp plain flour
1tsp hot smoked paprika
white bloomer or farmhouse loaf
mayonnaise
light oil, for frying
juice of roughly ½ lemon
lettuce (*optional*)
sea salt

Whitebait – tiny little fish perfect for frying and enjoying whole – are seriously underrated everywhere that is not the Great British Pub. You've probably seen them on the menu, gently spiced, fried and served with some sort of flavoured mayo for dipping. Here they are the answer to getting the perfect taste of the English seaside at home with a nice, hot sandwich that is a treat to eat, probably still standing over the stove.

1. Pat any excess water off the whitebait with kitchen paper. Mix together the flour and the paprika in a small bowl and toss together with the whitebait, making sure that they're all well coated.

2. Cut four thick slices of bread and spread two of them generously with mayonnaise.

3. Heat a medium frying pan over a high heat. Add enough oil to cover the bottom by about 5mm (¼in). Using a square of stale bread or a bit torn off the loaf, test the temperature of the oil; it should sizzle when dropped in the pan.

4. Fry the whitebait in batches for 3–4 minutes until golden on each side. Use a slotted spoon to transfer to a plate lined with kitchen paper to drain away any excess fat.

5. Pile the still hot whitebait on to the mayo-spread slices of bread, before sprinkling with a little sea salt and giving them a good spritz of fresh lemon. Add a little lettuce if you want before finishing the sandwich and enjoying right away.

tip

Whitebait tends to come ready-coated in breadcrumbs from the supermarket, but you should be able to get a big bag of frozen whitebait from most good fishmonger's.

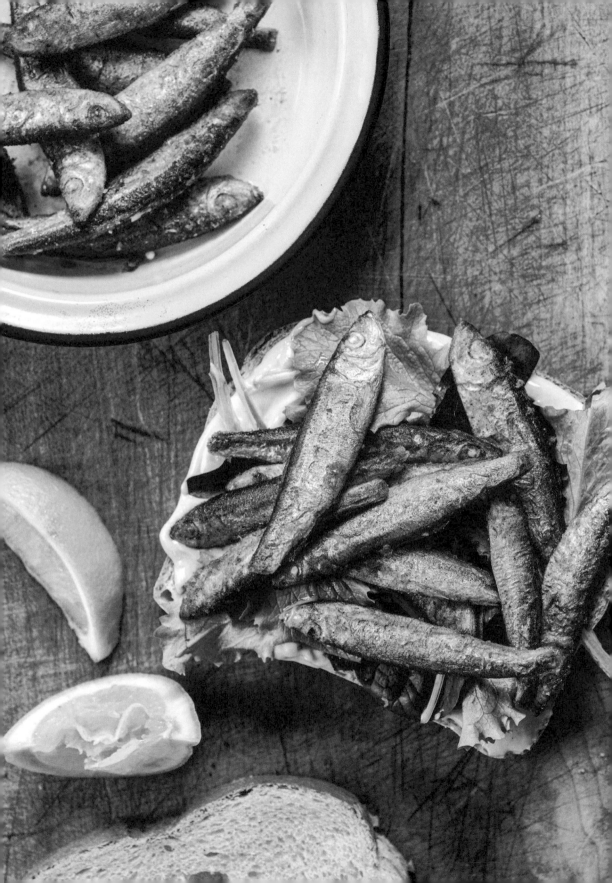

Lemony Garlic Butter Scallops with Tagliatelle

SERVES 2

Preparation time: 5 minutes
Cooking time: 30 minutes

200g (7oz) tagliatelle
unsalted butter, for frying
pinch of dried chilli flakes
2 large garlic cloves
8 fat scallops, roe removed
generous splash of white wine
small handful of fresh flat leaf
  parsley
sea salt and freshly ground black
  pepper

I know a lot of people are scared of cooking scallops at home (I know I certainly was) but after my dad made them for the first time – on my parents' wedding anniversary no less – without realising they were something he was supposed to be intimidated by and they came out perfectly, I realised most people's mistakes are because they're afraid of making a mistake. If you get all your ingredients prepared beforehand, however, scallops are actually pretty easy to get right.

1. In a large, shallow casserole dish big enough to lay down the tagliatelle in, cook the pasta in boiling salted water until tender – this should take 15 minutes but start testing the odd piece after 10 minutes.

2. Drain the pasta and set aside. Return the pan to a medium-high heat and add a very large knob of unsalted butter along with the chilli flakes and the garlic cloves, peeled and thinly sliced. Fry until the butter is melted and frothy.

3. Turn the heat up to high and season the scallops on both sides with salt and pepper. Place the scallops down in the butter and leave to cook for a minute or two, trying not to disturb them, until their bottoms are golden. Turn them over with a pair of tongs and cook until they're half a minute off being just as brown as they are on top.

4. Add the wine and allow it to bubble away. Return the pasta to the pan along with the parsley, roughly chopped, and another knob of butter. Stir until the pasta is well coated in the garlic butter sauce and check the seasoning.

5. Serve immediately in warm bowls, sitting four scallops on top of each bowl of tagliatelle.

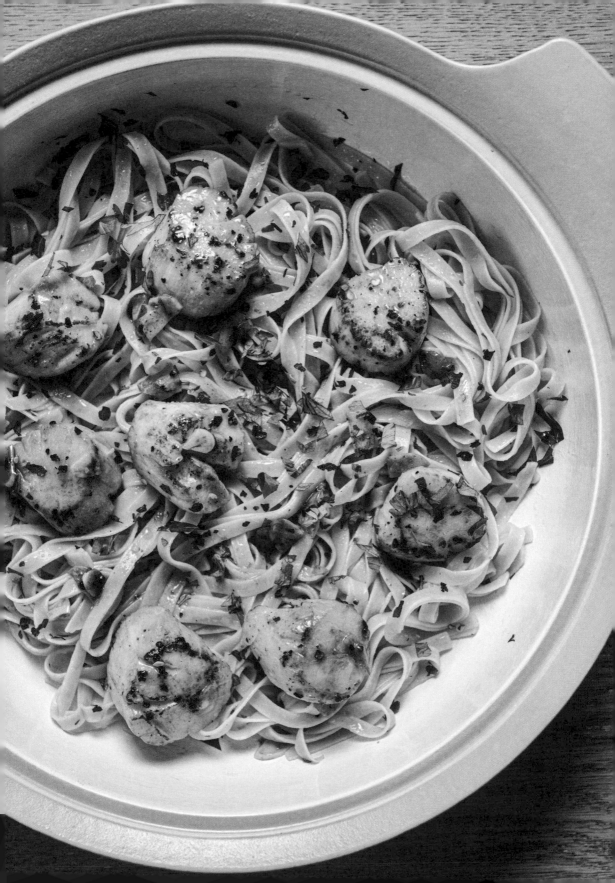

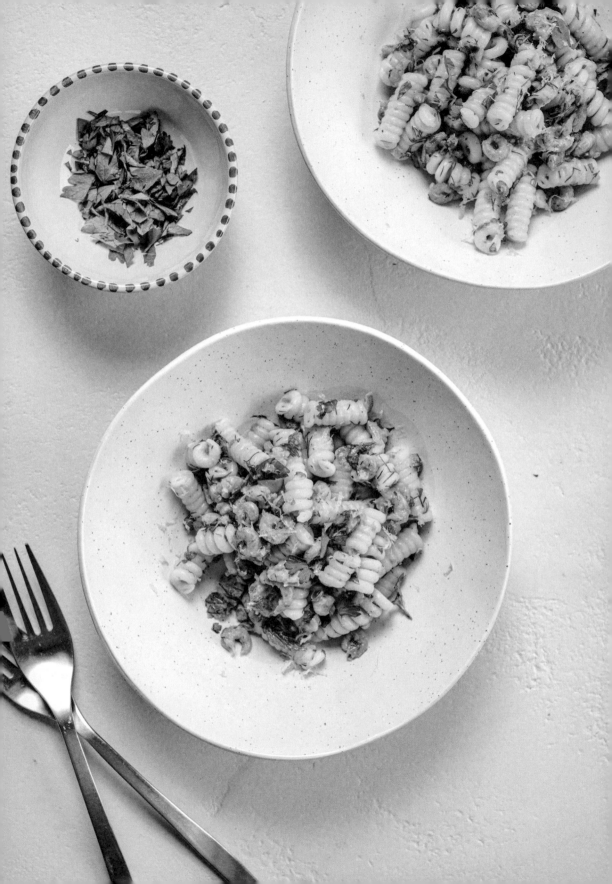

Pasta with Brown Shrimps

SERVES 2

Preparation time: 5 minutes
Cooking time: 20 minutes

200g (7oz) pasta shapes
2 tbsp non-pareille capers (see
   tip on page 172)
handful of fresh dill
handful of fresh flat leaf parsley
10 anchovy fillets, packed in oil
1 tbsp Dijon mustard
1 tsp extra virgin olive oil
zest of 1 lemon
200–300g (7–10oz) brown
   shrimps
freshly ground sea salt and black
   pepper

Mixing mustard into a bowl of pasta may sound a little strange, but with handfuls of fresh herbs, capers and sweet little brown shrimps it really works. Don't skimp on the anchovy here as it really is essential to adding a fishy little boost to the shrimps, which by themselves tend to be quite mild and delicate.

1. Cook the pasta in a saucepan of boiling, salted water as per the packet instructions. I find this usually takes around 15 minutes but start checking it after 10 minutes.

2 Meanwhile, roughly chop the capers and soft herbs and finely chop the anchovies.

3. Combine the capers, herbs and anchovies with the mustard, olive oil and lemon zest. Season well with salt and pepper and set aside.

4. Drain the pasta and return to the pan along with the caper mixture and the brown shrimps. Stir until everything is combined, then check the seasoning before serving.

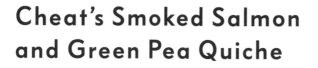

Cheat's Smoked Salmon and Green Pea Quiche

SERVES 4–6

Preparation time: 10 minutes
Cooking time: 45 minutes

unsalted butter, at room
  temperature
plain flour
1 × 320g (11oz) puff pastry sheet
150g (1 cup) frozen petit pois,
  defrosted
100g (3½oz) smoked salmon
100g (3½oz) pre-cooked salmon
2 large eggs
2 large egg yolks
150ml (⅔ cup) single cream
50ml (3 tbsp) milk
large handful of fresh dill
freshly ground sea salt and black
  pepper

tip

*You can find steamed or
poached salmon fillets in most
supermarkets, both work well in
this recipe. Or you can pre-cook
your own salmon in advance if
you prefer.*

This quiche is the result of what happened when my mum's recipe for a classic quiche Lorraine met a smoked salmon, potato and dill tart I made from *BBC Good Food Magazine* one Boxing Day to wide acclaim. It then morphed into an easy dinner party recipe that was among the first I wrote for Refinery 29. As with most of my favourite recipes I can never leave well alone, so now I bring you this third version, still as simple and foolproof to pull off as my previous one, but with the addition of pre-cooked salmon to add a little more interest and texture.

1. Preheat the oven to 200°C/400°F/Gas 6 and generously butter a round, shallow quiche or pie dish.

2. If your puff pastry sheet is a little wider at its narrowest point than your dish, great! If not, lightly dust a clean work surface with plain flour and roll the sheet out so that it is.

3. Lay the puff pastry sheet over the buttered dish and gently push it into the corners. Lift the dish slightly off the work surface for easy manoeuvring, then use a sharp knife to trim off the excess overhanging pastry.

4. Use your fingers to crimp/scallop the edges evenly all around.

5. Sprinkle the petit pois across the bottom of the pie case, followed by the smoked salmon, roughly torn, and the cooked salmon, flaked into bite-sized chunks.

6. In a mixing jug, whisk together the eggs, egg yolks, cream, milk and the dill, finely chopped, along with a generous amount of salt and pepper until the mixture is uniform.

7. Pour the quiche mix over the fillings and transfer the dish to the oven for 40–45 minutes. You'll know it is done when the

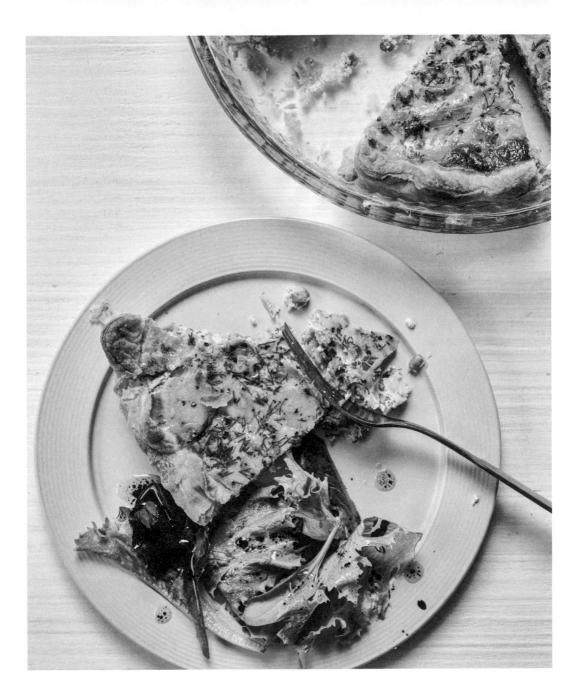

pastry is crisp and golden, and the quiche filling has also browned, set, and puffed up a little.

8. Leave the quiche for at least 10 minutes before slicing, I always think it tastes best served at room temperature.

Devilled Crab Gnocchi

SERVES 2

Preparation time: 5 minutes
Cooking time: 5 minutes

500g (1lb 2oz) gnocchi
2 large spring onions
300g (10oz) mixed crabmeat
½ tsp Worcestershire sauce
10–12 dashes of Tabasco
juice of roughly ¼ lemon
small handful of fresh flat leaf
  parsley
freshly ground sea salt and black
  pepper

I created this quick, easy and indulgent devilled crab gnocchi as a response to some leftover brown crab meat I had in the fridge from making a crab, chilli and courgette dish. It's super-rich, very comforting and slightly spicy. To lighten things up a bit, I'd serve it with a light green salad with lots of spring onions to cut through the sauce and a nice fruity glass of red wine.

1. Cook the gnocchi in a large saucepan of boiling water. This only takes a couple of minutes – you can tell it is done when the gnocchi starts to float to the surface of the pan.

2. Meanwhile, make the sauce by thinly slicing the spring onions and combining them with the crabmeat, Worcestershire sauce, Tabasco and a generous amount of salt and pepper in a large bowl. Season to taste with fresh lemon juice and more salt, if needed.

3. Drain the gnocchi well and fold them into the crab mixture. Roughly chop the parsley and sprinkle over the top before serving.

Orange and Rosemary Marinated Fish with Courgette Salad

SERVES 2

Preparation time: 15 minutes
Cooking time: 5 minutes

1 garlic clove
1 small orange
1 red chilli
2½ tbsp extra virgin olive oil
1 tsp finely chopped fresh
   rosemary
2 large fillets of sustainable sea
   bass or other thin fillets of white
   fish
1 large courgette
freshly ground sea salt and black
   pepper

I'd recommend cooking this over a charcoal barbecue, but I've also cooked it in a griddle pan with good results. I've used sea bass fillets here as they're easy for most people to get, but feel free to use any other fillet of white fish. This is a really light, fresh meal, so do feel free to serve it with some crusty bread or some buttered, boiled new potatoes.

1. To make the marinade for the fish, peel and crush the garlic clove and combine it in a shallow dish with the zest of quarter of the orange, half the chilli (deseeded and finely chopped), 2 tablespoons of the oil, the rosemary and a good amount of salt and pepper. Add the fish fillets, flesh side down, and leave them to marinate.

2. To make the courgette salad, use a vegetable peeler to cut the courgette into thin ribbons and toss together with a good few grinds of sea salt in a medium bowl. Peel and cut the orange into segments and add them to the bowl along with the remaining chilli, thinly sliced, and the remaining olive oil. Set aside.

3. Cook the fish, first skin side down until crisp, then flesh side down until lines just start to appear and the flesh is flaky and tender. Do this over the hottest part of the barbecue or in a very hot griddle pan. Be careful, sea bass can be delicate, but I think that is part of its charm!

4. Serve the grilled fish with the raw courgette salad alongside.

Spring Pea Risotto with Fresh Crab

SERVES 2

Preparation time: 15 minutes
Cooking time: 50 minutes

4 crab claws
1 small onion
1 tbsp light oil
150g (¾ cup) risotto rice
130ml (½ cup) white wine
770ml (3¼ cups) hot vegetable
  stock
100g (⅔ cup) frozen petit pois
small knob unsalted butter
zest of ½ lemon
freshly ground sea salt and black
  pepper

I have so much love for this risotto. Light and elegant, with fresh peas and great chunks of fresh crab meat, it is probably the most sophisticated recipe in the book. I've given some more notes on cooking risotto on pages 60–62 so do check there first, especially if you prefer to make your risotto in a wide, shallow casserole as I did in that recipe, rather than in a big saucepan as I have done here.

1. Remove the meat from the crab claws (see tip), trying to keep as many chunks of crab meat intact as possible.

2. Heat a large saucepan over a medium heat. Peel and finely chop the onion and gently fry it in the oil, along with a large pinch of sea salt, until soft and lightly browned – this should take about 10 minutes.

3. Stir in the risotto rice until the grains have heated through, then add the wine and allow it to bubble away.

4. Reduce the heat to medium-low and gradually ladle the stock into the rice a spoonful at a time, stirring almost continuously, until you've used up all the stock and the rice is plump, thick and almost tender.

5. Season well with black pepper and check to see if you'd like to add any more salt. Add the frozen petit pois and cook for a further 5 minutes until they are heated through.

6. Stir in the lemon zest and a small knob of unsalted butter. Carefully fold in the crab meat, doing your best not to break up the lumps and reserving a few choice pieces to scatter on top of each dish before serving.

tip

You can usually find crab claws on supermarket fish counters or fishmongers. They might come with the shells ready-scored but if not wrap them in a clean tea towel before hitting with a hammer.

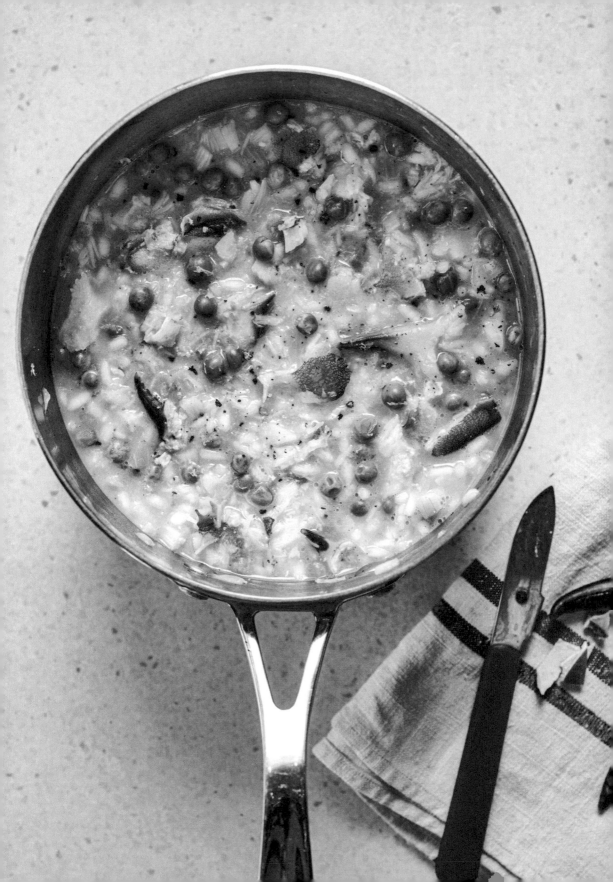

Flash-fried Squid with Chickpeas, Tomatoes and Romesco

SERVES 2

Preparation time: 10 minutes
Cooking time: 15 minutes

The star of this summertime plateful of flashy flavours is this vibrant romesco sauce. I like to make up a massive jar full of the stuff and keep it in the fridge to serve with as many things I can get away with.

For the romesco sauce
200g (7oz) jarred roasted
  peppers in brine
small handful of blanched
  almonds
1 tbsp extra virgin olive oil
2 tsp sherry vinegar
½ tsp sweet smoked paprika
large pinch of sea salt

For the flash-fried squid
400g (14oz) tin chickpeas
small handful of flat leaf parsley
1½ tbsp extra virgin olive oil
juice of roughly ½ lemon
300g (1½ cups) cherry tomatoes
2 large squid, cleaned
freshly ground sea salt and black
  pepper

1. First, make the romesco sauce. Drain, deseed and chop the peppers before adding them to a high-speed blender or food processor with the rest of the ingredients. Blitz until smooth, then check the seasoning. Set aside.

2. To prepare the chickpeas, drain and rinse off any excess liquid. Pat dry on a piece of kitchen paper and combine with the parsley (roughly chopped) half a tablespoon of the olive oil, a good squeeze of lemon juice and a generous amount of salt and pepper.

3. Heat another half tablespoon of oil in a large frying pan over a high heat. Halve the cherry tomatoes and toss them into the pan, seasoning well and quickly frying them until they just start to blister and char. Remove and set aside.

4. Wipe the pan clean using another piece of kitchen paper and add the remaining tablespoon of oil. Slice the squid into thick chunks, scoring each in a hatch pattern to get a good char, but making sure not to cut all the way through the flesh. Season the squid with salt and pepper and add it to the pan in a single layer, cut side down. When it starts to curl, turn the pieces over to colour the other side.

5. When the squid is just cooked but still tender, return the cherry tomatoes to the pan and toss until warmed through.

6. To serve, divide the chickpeas between two bowls and top with the squid and tomato mixture. Serve the romesco sauce in a little bowl on the side, for drizzling.

tip

My favourite ways to use romesco are: spooned over a plate of griddled veggies and brown rice, dolloped on the side of some chunky roasted leeks and skin on chicken thighs, or simply as a condiment to a roast chicken.

Californian Seafood Stew

SERVES 2

Preparation time: 10 minutes
Cooking time: 40 minutes

generous splash of light oil
1 small onion
1 large celery stick
3 large garlic cloves
1 dried bay leaf
2 tsp rose harissa
150ml (⅔ cup) dry white wine
400g (14oz) tin cherry or
   chopped tomatoes
125g (4½oz) white fish fillets
   (*I use bream*)
6 large shell-on king prawns
400g (14oz) mussels
2 large slices of sourdough bread
small handful of fresh flat leaf
   parsley
freshly ground sea salt and black
   pepper

Tomato-based stews, heavy with the local catch that flavours the broth, are common across the Mediterranean, but here I'm taking inspiration from San Francisco's 'cioppino' stew, served with a couple of nicely toasted shards of garlicky sourdough on the side for dunking.

1. Heat the oil over a medium-high heat in a large, lidded saucepan. Peel and finely chop the onion and top, tail and finely chop the celery. Fry together with a large pinch of sea salt for 5 minutes or so until tender and just starting to colour.

2. Peel and thinly slice two of the garlic cloves and add them to the pan, frying for another minute or so until aromatic. Add the bay leaf and the harissa and fry for another minute.

3. Add the wine and allow the alcohol to bubble away for another minute or so before adding the tinned tomatoes and 250ml water. Season well with black pepper and turn the heat up to high. Once bubbling, turn it down to low and allow to simmer, uncovered, for 20 minutes.

4. Cut the fish into bite-sized pieces – leaving the skin on will stop them breaking down entirely into the stew (you'll be fishing mussel shells out anyway) and add them to the pan along with the prawns and mussels, cleaned and de-bearded (see page 161). Put on the lid and leave to simmer for 4–5 minutes until the fish is cooked through, the prawns have gone from grey to a beautiful, sun-drenched orange, and the mussels shells have just opened.

5. Meanwhile, toast the sourdough, and halve the remaining garlic clove – don't worry about peeling it. Rub the garlic over each half of toast and set aside.

6. Divide the stew between two bowls, discarding any unopened mussels. Roughly chop the parsley and sprinkle generously on top. Serve the garlic bread half dunked into each bowl of stew.

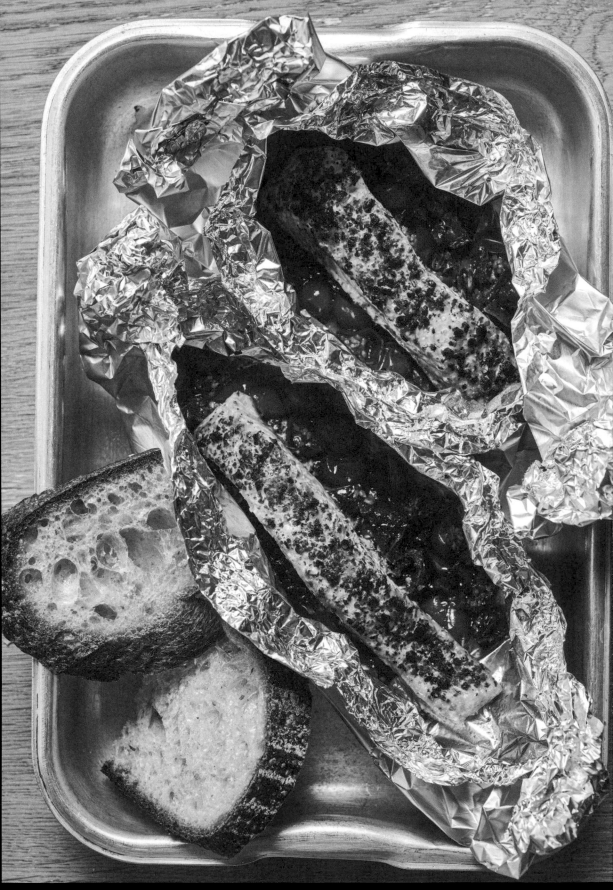

Mediterranean Salmon Parcels

SERVES 1 OR MORE

Preparation time: 5 minutes
Cooking time: 30 minutes

Per portion
100g (½ cup) cherry tomatoes
1 tbsp sun-dried tomatoes,
    packed in oil
1 salmon fillet
1 tsp extra virgin olive oil
½ tsp Aleppo chilli flakes
freshly ground sea salt and black
    pepper

It sounds simple but a piece of salmon baked in tin foil is one of mine and my mum's favourite dinners to enjoy together when I'm home. I've made this Mediterranean-inspired version a single serving because you do have to cook each portion individually, but feel free to scale it up to feed as many people as you like! I like this – as always – served with lots of crusty bread to mop up the cooking juices, but some brown rice would also work well.

1. Preheat the oven to 200°C/400°F/Gas 6. Lay out one large piece of foil per portion of fish.

2 Halve the cherry tomatoes, roughly chop the sun-dried tomatoes and place them in the middle of the foil. Lay the salmon fillet, skin side down, on top and drizzle with the olive oil. Season well with salt and pepper and sprinkle the top of the salmon with Aleppo chilli flakes.

3. Gather the sides of the foil up around the salmon and the tomatoes to make a little boat, then fold and scrunch the foil at the top and at both ends to create a sealed packet. Try to leave as much room for the salmon to steam as possible while keeping it sealed. Transfer the parcels to a baking tray.

4. Bake the salmon packet for about 30 minutes until the salmon is just cooked – it should be tender and flaky, but still slightly pink in the middle.

Barbecued Mackerel with Cucumber and Chilli Salad

SERVES 2

Preparation time: 15 minutes
Cooking time: 20 minutes

This is one of those super-light summertime suppers you really do need the barbecue for. I find this filling enough but if you're craving some carbs, brown basmati rice is a good addition, drizzled with some soy sauce.

For the mackerel
juice of 1 lime
1 tbsp freshly grated ginger
large pinch of golden caster
   sugar
4 mackerel fillets
freshly ground sea salt and black
   pepper

For the gem lettuce
2 gem lettuces
2 tsp fish sauce

**For the cucumber and
chilli salad**
1 large cucumber
1 red chilli
2 tsp rice wine vinegar
½ tbsp fresh ginger, grated on the
   large hole of the box grater
½ tsp sea salt
¼ tsp golden caster sugar

1. Combine the lime juice, ginger, sugar and a generous amount of salt and pepper in a shallow dish. Place the mackerel fillets flesh side down in the marinade and set aside while you light the barbecue. You want a high heat in the middle, with cooler space around the edge to keep cooked food warm.

2. Halve the gem lettuces down the middle, discarding any soft or crushed leaves. Drizzle the cut side of each half with ½ teaspoon of fish sauce.

3. To make the cucumber salad, peel the cucumber, cut it into quarters and place it in a plastic bag. Deseed and thinly slice the chilli before adding it to the bag along with the vinegar, ginger, salt and sugar. Tie a knot in the end and use a rolling pin to lightly smash the cucumber until you get just slightly larger than bite-sized chunks. Set aside.

4. Once the barbecue is hot, char the lettuces, cut side down, for 3–4 minutes until coloured. Turn cut side up and move them to the cooler edge of your cooking area to wilt.

5. Remove the mackerel from the marinade and place it skin side down in the middle of the heat, drizzling with any leftover marinade. Cook for about 4–5 minutes until the skin has started to bubble and crisp, then flip the fish over and cook for a further 3–4 minutes until cooked through and charred a little on each side.

6. Serve the fish and lettuce with the cucumber salad on the side with a little of the cucumber marinade drizzled over.

Korean Salmon with Sesame Veggies

SERVES 2

Preparation time: 15 minutes
Cooking time: 30 minutes

For the salmon
1 large garlic clove
1½ tbsp gochujang
½ tbsp maple syrup
splash of toasted sesame oil
2 salmon fillets
furikake, to serve

For the sesame veggies
2 pak choi
3 tsp toasted sesame oil
1 tsp fish sauce
1 courgette
½ tsp golden caster sugar
½ tsp rice wine vinegar
½ tsp soy sauce
½ tsp gochugaru
4 large spring onions
80g (¾ cup) sugar snap peas

This sticky Korean-flavoured salmon dish is inspired by one of my favourite packed lunches. I used to double the sticky, tender salmon and cook rice to pack up with some chopped cucumber and an Asian-inspired dressing in a little squeezy bottle. This is the version I make when I'm not worried about having enough leftovers for lunch the next day.

1. Preheat the oven to 200°C/400°F/Gas 6. Start by making the salmon marinade. Whisk together the garlic clove, peeled and crushed, the gochujang, maple syrup and sesame oil to form a thick paste. Coat the salmon fillets and set aside.

2. Remove the soft, leafy green tops from the pak choi and set aside. Halve the bulbs down the middle, placing them cut side up on a large baking tray. Drizzle the cut halves with 2 teaspoons of the toasted sesame oil (reserving the remaining 1 teaspoon for later), and do the same with the fish sauce.

3. Roughly chop the courgette into half-moons and toss them with a further ½ teaspoon of sesame oil on the baking tray alongside the pak choi. Transfer to the oven to roast for 15 minutes.

4. Meanwhile, make the spring onion salad. In a small bowl, whisk together the sugar, vinegar, soy sauce, gochugaru and the remaining ½ teaspoon of sesame oil. Set aside. Trim the spring onions and slice them into thin strips. Shred the reserved pak choi into 5mm (¼in) ribbons and set aside.

5. Toss the sugar snap peas together with the courgette on the baking tray and add the salmon, skin side down. Roast for a further 10–15 minutes until the salmon is just cooked: flaky, but still a little pink in the middle. Serve the salmon alongside the roasted veggies, with the raw salad, tossed in the dressing at the last minute. Sprinkle a little furikake over each salmon fillet before bringing it to the table.

Thai Prawn, Avocado, Red Rice and Mango Bowl

SERVES 4

Preparation time: 10 minutes
Cooking time: 30 minutes

220g (generous 1 cup) red rice
200g (7oz) cooked king prawns
2 large ripe avocados
400g (14oz) ripe mango
large handful of fresh chives

For the dressing
2 tbsp sweet chilli sauce
4 tsp fish sauce
2 tsp fresh lime juice
1 tsp fresh grated ginger

I like to use red rice as I love the colour and nuttiness it lends to rice salads (I buy it from health-food shops but you can always use brown basmati if you can't find it); paired with refreshing mango and creamy avocado, this salad is a textural dream.

1. Cook the rice in a saucepan of boiling water for 25–35 minutes. The rice is ready when the kernels start to pop open and reveal their soft middles. I always cook my rice like pasta, in a pan of water and drain it rather than using the absorption method – that way is the quickest and easiest way to burn rice. Drain the rice using a sieve, then run it under a cold tap and set aside to continue draining. If you're making this ahead, leave the rice to cool, but remember rice left out too long on the countertop can start to grow harmful bacteria!

2. Meanwhile, pat the prawns dry of any excess liquid on a piece of kitchen paper and halve down the middle to create two smaller prawn chunks. Transfer these to a large bowl along with the avocado, peeled and cut into slightly smaller than bite-sized cubes, the mango, cut likewise, and the chives, snipped into very small pieces with a pair of kitchen scissors.

3. To make the dressing, whisk together the sweet chilli sauce, fish sauce, lime juice and ginger.

4. Carefully fold the rice and half the dressing into the bowl until everything is combined, working carefully so not to bash up the avocado too much. Add the rest of the dressing to taste but make sure you don't make the salad too wet - this will depend on how much excess moisture remains in your rice.

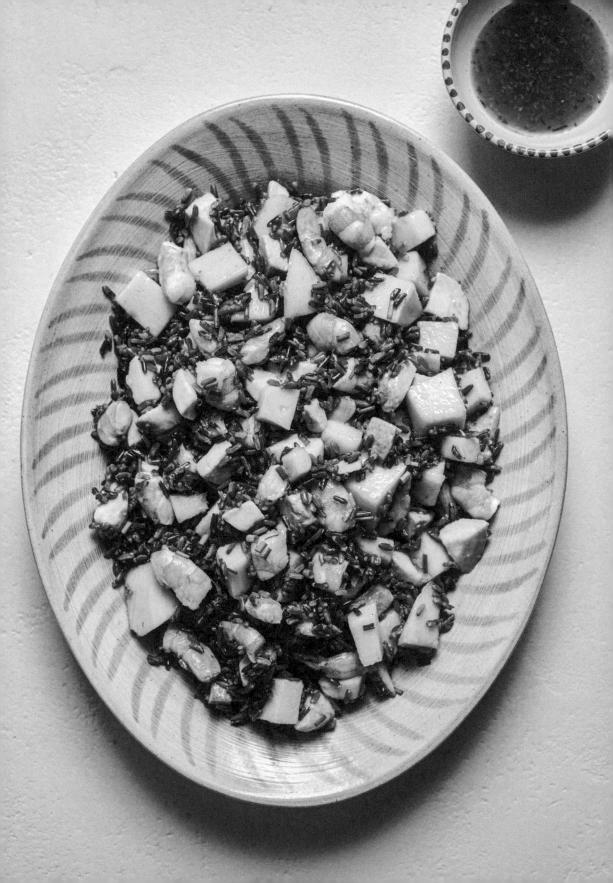

Index

A

almond 210
   California kale, orange, almond and
      mushroom salad 112–13, *113*
   dukkah spaghetti with raw tomato
      and almond sauce 136, *137*
   tomato, almond and thyme tart
      34, 35
anchovy 178
   anchovy butter 170–1, *171*
asparagus
   asparagus and goats' curd pancake
      56, 57
aubergine 142
   roast aubergine and fresh tomato
      salad with basil vinaigrette 118, *119*
avocado 28, 65, 115, 122, 164, 190
   cured salmon avocado toast 160
   Thai prawn, avocado, red rice and
      mango bowl 216, *217*
   watermelon, avocado and feta
      salad with lime dressing 68, 69

B

banchan 74–5
barbeques 12, 116, 214
basil 26, 36, 70, 117, 132, 133, 163
   baked gnocchi with tomatoes, basil
      and marinated mozzarella 40, *41*
   pasta shells with fresh tomato, crab
      and basil 188
   roast aubergine and fresh tomato
      salad with basil vinaigrette 118, *119*
   tomato, basil and feta orzotto 38
bean(s)
   gigantes plaki with feta 70
   slow cooker mixed bean chilli 126, *127*
   tomato braised bean and white fish
      stew with gremolata *176*, 177
   see also black bean
beetroot and dill cured salmon 158–9,
   159

black bean 28, 65, 124, 131, 180
   slow cooker mixed bean chilli 126
blinis, homemade blini pancakes 160
bread 39, 47, 80, 120, 194, 211
   cacio e pepe eggy bread crumpets
      58, *59*
   tomato, black olive and courgette
      bread with anchovy butter
      170–1, *171*
broccoli *see* Tenderstem broccoli
bruschetta, white peach, mozzarella
   and pea shoot bruschetta 39
Brussels sprout, warm roasted sprout
   salad with pecorino and pear 30, *31*
burgers, pea and courgette burgers
   with kimchee 78, *79*
butter
   anchovy butter 170–1, *171*
   lemony garlic butter 200, *201*
butternut squash 102
   creamy butternut squash risotto
      60, *61–3*

C

Cajun seasoning
   Cajun salmon traybake with
      tropical fruit salsa 180, *181*
   crispy Cajun coconut prawn tacos
      182, 183
carrot 80, 96–8, 99, 102, 132
casserole, tomato and root veggie
   casserole with herby dumplings
   96–8, *97*
cauliflower, roasted sweet potato and
   cauliflower hummus bowls 104, *105*
celery 99, 132, 177, 211
chaat salad 88, *89*
chickpeas 88
   dhal baked eggs with chickpeas
      90–1, *91*
   flash-fried squid with chickpeas,
      tomatoes and romesco 210

hummus toast with tomatoes,
   chickpeas and crispy kale 120
sheet pan chickpea fajitas 128, *129*
tomato and chickpea alphabet
   soup 66, 67
chilli, slow cooker mixed bean chilli
   126, *127*
chipotle
   creamy sweetcorn and chipotle
      soup 125
   honey chipotle dressing 28, *29*
chips, fancy Friday night fish and chips
   196, 197
ciabatta, feta, muhammara
   and charred broccoli ciabatta
   sandwiches 42, *43*
coconut 151
   coconut curry zoodles with Asian
      greens and silken tofu 82, *83*
   crispy Cajun coconut prawn tacos
      183
cod
   black olive tapenade cod with
      summer vegetables 184, *185*
   fancy Friday night fish and chips
      197
   tomato braised bean and white fish
      stew with gremolata 177
courgette 37, 82, 138, 142, 146, 215
   easy summertime courgette soup
      140, 141
   fried courgettes on toast with
      ricotta and fresh herbs 46, *47*
   orange and rosemary marinated
      fish with courgette salad 207
   pea and courgette burgers with
      kimchee 78, *79*
   tomato, black olive and courgette
      bread with anchovy butter
      170–1, *171*
   tomato and courgette baked
      eggs 36

crab
    devilled crab gnocchi 206
    pasta shells with fresh tomato, crab
        and basil 188
    spring pea risotto with fresh crab
        208, *209*
crayfish, classic crayfish rolls 194, *195*
crumpets, cacio e pepe eggy bread
    crumpets 58, *59*
cucumber 156
    barbecued mackerel with
        cucumber and chilli salad 214
    Korean cucumber pickles 115
    spicy cucumber and silken tofu rice
        noodles 148, *149*
curry, coconut curry zoodles with Asian
    greens and silken tofu 82, *83*

D

dhal
    dhal baked eggs with chickpeas
        90–1, *91*
    dhal makhani 86, *87*
dressings 216
    honey chipotle dressing 28, *29*
    lime dressing 68, *69*
    maple mustard dressing 102, *103*
dukkah spaghetti with raw tomato and
    almond sauce 136, *137*
dumplings, tomato and root veggie
    casserole with herby dumplings
    96–8, *97*

E

egg 24, 35, 48, 57, 76, 78, 85, 178, 183,
    186, 190, 204–5
    cacio e pepe eggy bread crumpets
        58
    dhal baked eggs with chickpeas
        90–1, *91*
    Mexican baked eggs 65
    spinach, egg and mushroom Dutch
        baby pancake 54–5, *55*

tomato and courgette baked
    eggs 36
    Turk-ish baked eggs 44, *45*

F

fajitas, sheet pan chickpea fajitas 128,
    129
fennel, whole roast sea bass with
    fennel and potatoes 174, *175*
feta 42, 44, 73, 163
    feta, veggie and lemon bake 26, *27*
    gigantes plaki with feta 70, *71*
    roasted red pepper, spring onion
        and feta frittata 48
    tomato, basil and feta orzotto 38
    watermelon, avocado and feta
        salad with lime dressing 68, *69*
fish 8, 153–217
fish and chips, fancy Friday night fish
    and chips 196, *197*
French onion soup with goats' cheese
    toasts 64
frittata, roasted red pepper, spring
    onion and feta frittata 48
fritters, courgette, lemon and ricotta
    fritters 37
furikake 16, 85, 115, 144, 146, 156, 164,
    215

G

garlic
    garlicky moules with tiny pasta 189
    hot prawns in garlic butter 166, *167*
    lemony garlic butter scallops with
        tagliatelle 200, *201*
gnocchi
    baked gnocchi with tomatoes, basil
        and marinated mozzarella 40, *41*
    devilled crab gnocchi 206
    summer veggie crispy gnocchi
        bake 32, *33*
goats' cheese, French onion soup with
    goats' cheese toasts 64

gochugaru 16, 115, 215
gochujang 15, 75, 76, 146, 156, 215
gremolata *176*, 177

H

honey chipotle dressing 28, *29*
hummus
    deli counter hummus pasta 117
    hummus toast with tomatoes,
        chickpeas and crispy kale 120
    roasted sweet potato and
        cauliflower hummus bowls
        104, *105*

K

kale
    California kale, orange, almond
        and mushroom salad 112–13, *113*
    hummus toast with tomatoes,
        chickpeas and crispy kale 120
kedgeree, one pan smoked salmon
    kedgeree 186, *187*
Kewpie mayonnaise 16–17, 73, 78, 80
kimchee 15, 75
    easy salmon poke bowls 164
    kimchee fried rice 9, *76*, *77*
    pea and courgette burgers with
        kimchee 78, *79*

L

leek 96–8
    velvet vegan leek and potato soup
        100, *101*
lemon
    courgette, lemon and ricotta
        fritters 37
    feta, veggie and lemon bake 26, *27*
    green pea and lemon pesto
        pasta 133
    lemon pesto 132
    lemony garlic butter scallops with
        tagliatelle 200, *201*
lentil(s) 86, 90–1, 108

lime dressing 68, 69

M

mackerel, barbecued mackerel with cucumber and chilli salad 214

mango, Thai prawn, avocado, red rice and mango bowl 216, *217*

maple mustard dressing 102, *103*

minestrone soup 132

miso, sweet potato miso soup 144, *145*

molasses 17, 42, 104

    tomato salad with pomegranate molasses 121

mozzarella

    baked gnocchi with tomatoes, basil and marinated mozzarella 40, *41*

    white peach, mozzarella and pea shoot bruschetta 39

muhammara

    feta, muhammara and charred broccoli ciabatta sandwiches 42, *43*

    spaghetti with muhammara sauce *106*, 107

mushroom

    California kale, orange, almond and mushroom salad 112–13, *113*

    savoury wild mushroom oatmeal 49

    spinach, egg and mushroom Dutch baby pancake 54–5, *55*

mushy peas 197

mussel(s) 211

    Cornish mussels 161

    garlicky moules with tiny pasta 189

mustard, maple mustard dressing 102, *103*

N

noodle(s)

    slow cooker ramen *84*, 85

    spicy cucumber and silken tofu rice noodles 148, *149*

O

oat(s)

    savoury wild mushroom oatmeal 49

spinach and oatmeal pancakes 190, *191*

oils 14

olive (black) 26, 117

    black olive tapenade cod with summer vegetables 184, *185*

    tomato, black olive and courgette bread with anchovy butter 170–1, *171*

onion

    French onion soup with goats' cheese toasts 64

    plantain tacos with quick pickled onions and smashed avocado 122, *123*

orange

    California kale, orange, almond and mushroom salad 112–13, *113*

    orange and rosemary marinated fish with courgette salad 207

orzo, tomato, basil and feta orzotto 38

P

paella, veggie paella 138, *139*

pak choi 82, 85, 215

pancakes

    homemade blini pancakes 160

    spinach, egg and mushroom Dutch baby pancake 54–5, *55*

    spinach and oatmeal pancakes 190, *191*

Parmesan 32, 49, 50–2, 54–5, 58, 60, 66

parsnip 96–8

passata 50–2, 86, 90–1, 142

pasta

    alphabet minestrone soup 132

    deli counter hummus pasta 117

    dukkah spaghetti with raw tomato and almond sauce 136, *137*

    garlicky moules with tiny pasta 189

    green pea and lemon pesto pasta 133

    lemony garlic butter scallops with tagliatelle 200, *201*

    pasta with brown shrimps *202*, 203

    pasta shells with fresh tomato, crab and basil 188

smoked salmon spaghetti 192, *193*

spaghetti with muhammara sauce *106*, 107

spinach and ricotta stuffed shells in tomato sauce 50–2, *51–3*

tomato, basil and feta orzotto 38

tomato and chickpea alphabet soup 66

ultimate tuna pasta 172, *173*

peach, white peach, mozzarella and pea shoot bruschetta 39

pear, warm roasted sprout salad with pecorino and pear 30, *31*

pea(s) 186

    cheat's smoked salmon and green pea quiche 204–5, *205*

    green pea and lemon pesto pasta 133

    mushy peas 197

    pea and courgette burgers with kimchee 78, *79*

    spring pea risotto with fresh crab 208, *209*

    Thai green pea soup *150*, 151

pecorino 32

    warm roasted sprout salad with pecorino and pear 30, *31*

pepper 26, 32, 42, 117, 126, 128, 138, 180, 184, 210

    roasted red pepper, spring onion and feta frittata 48

    sweet chilli and pepper barbecue tofu skewers 116

pesto, lemon pesto 132

pickles

    Korean cucumber pickles 115

    Vietnamese pickles 80

pine nut(s) 47, 132

plantain tacos with quick pickled onions and smashed avocado 122, *123*

pomegranate molasses, tomato salad with pomegranate molasses 121

pomegranate seeds 30, 42, 88, 104, 108, 118

potato 48, 88, 141, 178, 184

    fancy Friday night fish and chips 197

tomato and root veggie casserole with herby dumplings 96–8

velvet vegan leek and potato soup 100, *101*

whole roast sea bass with fennel and potatoes 174, *175*

prawn

California seafood stew 211

crispy Cajun coconut prawn tacos *182*, 183

hot prawns in garlic butter 166, *167*

prawn saganaki *162*, 163

Thai prawn, avocado, red rice and mango bowl 216, *217*

puff pastry

cheat's smoked salmon and green pea quiche 204–5

tomato, almond and thyme tart 35

Q

quiche, cheat's smoked salmon and green pea quiche 204–5, *205*

R

radish 80, 156, 164

ramen noodles, slow cooker ramen *84*, 85

ratatouille, easy ratatouille spiral 142, *143*

rice

creamy butternut squash risotto 60, *61–3*

easy salmon poke bowls 164, *165*

kimchee fried rice 9, 76, 77

Korean sashimi salad (*hwe dup bap*) 156

one pan smoked salmon kedgeree 186

spicy, herby two pouch mujadara 108, *109*

spring pea risotto with fresh crab 208, *209*

Thai prawn, avocado, red rice and mango bowl 216, *217*

vegan watermelon poke bowls *114*, 115

veggie paella 138, *139*

rice cakes, spicy Korean rice cakes (*Tteokbokki*) 146, *147*

rice noodles, spicy cucumber and

silken tofu rice noodles 148, *149*

ricotta

courgette, lemon and ricotta fritters 37

fried courgettes on toast with ricotta and fresh herbs 46, 47

spinach and ricotta stuffed shells in tomato sauce 50–2, *51–3*

risotto

creamy butternut squash risotto 60, *61–3*

spring pea risotto with fresh crab 208, *209*

romesco, flash-fried squid with chickpeas, tomatoes and romesco 210

S

saganaki, prawn saganaki *162*, 163

salads

barbecued mackerel with cucumber and chilli salad 214

California kale, orange, almond and mushroom salad 112–13, *113*

cheat's chaat salad 88, 89

grilled Mexican street corn salad *72*, 73

Korean sashimi salad (*hwe dup bap*) 156, *157*

Mexican roasted sweet potato salad with honey chipotle dressing 28, 29

orange and rosemary marinated fish with courgette salad 207

roast aubergine and fresh tomato salad with basil vinaigrette 118, *119*

tomato salad with pomegranate molasses 121

warm roasted sprout salad with pecorino and pear 30, *31*

watermelon, avocado and feta salad with lime dressing 68, 69

salmon

beetroot and dill cured salmon 158–9, *159*

Cajun salmon traybake with tropical fruit salsa 180, *181*

cheat's smoked salmon and green

pea quiche 204–5

cured salmon avocado toast 160

easy salmon poke bowls 164, *165*

Korean salmon with sesame veggies 215

Korean sashimi salad (*hwe dup bap*) 156

Mediterranean salmon parcels *212*, 213

one pan smoked salmon kedgeree 186, *187*

salmon (smoked)

cheat's smoked salmon and green pea quiche 204–5, *205*

smoked salmon spaghetti 192, *193*

spinach and oatmeal pancakes 190

salsa 124

Cajun salmon traybake with tropical fruit salsa 180, *181*

salsa verde 178, *179*

salt 14, 18, 168–9

whole baked fish in a sea salt crust 178, *179*

sandwiches

feta, muhammara and charred broccoli ciabatta sandwiches *42*, *43*

fried whitebait sandwich 198, *199*

tofu bánh mì sandwich 80, *81*

sashimi, Korean sashimi salad (*hwe dup bap*) 156, *157*

scallops, lemony garlic butter scallops with tagliatelle 200, *201*

sea bass

orange and rosemary marinated fish with courgette salad 207

whole baked fish in a sea salt crust 178

whole roast sea bass with fennel and potatoes 174, *175*

sea bream, whole baked fish in a sea salt crust 178

seafood, Californian seafood stew 211

seaweed, wakame seaweed salad 115

shrimp, pasta with brown shrimps *202*, 203

slow cookers 11, 85, 99, 126, 131

soup
alphabet minestrone soup 132
creamy sweetcorn and chipotle
soup 125
easy summertime courgette soup
140, 141
French onion soup with goats'
cheese toasts 64
slow cooker spicy tortilla soup *130*,
131
sweet potato miso soup 144, *145*
Thai green pea soup *150*, 151
tomato and chickpea alphabet
soup 66, 67
velvet vegan leek and potato soup
100, *101*
spinach 28
spinach, egg and mushroom Dutch
baby pancake 54–5, *55*
spinach and oatmeal pancakes
190, *191*
spinach and ricotta stuffed shells in
tomato sauce 50–2, *51–3*
spring onion 76, 82, 85, 115, 144, 146,
156, 206, 215
roasted red pepper, spring onion
and feta frittata 48
squid, flash-fried squid with chickpeas,
tomatoes and romesco 210
stew
Californian seafood stew 211
tomato braised bean and white fish
stew with gremolata *176*, 177
stock, slow cooker vegetable stock 99
sugar snap pea 82, 215
sustainability issues 8, 9
swede 96–8
sweet chilli sauce
Korean sweet chilli sauce 156
sweet chilli and pepper barbecue
tofu skewers 116
sweet potato 102
Mexican roasted sweet potato
salad with honey chipotle
dressing 28, *29*
roasted sweet potato and
cauliflower hummus bowls
104, *105*

sweet potato miso soup 144, *145*
sweetcorn
creamy sweetcorn and chipotle
soup 125
grilled Mexican street corn salad
72, 73

T

tacos
crispy Cajun coconut prawn tacos
182, 183
plantain tacos with quick pickled
onions and smashed avocado
122, *123*
tapenade, black olive tapenade cod
with summer vegetables 184, *185*
tart, tomato, almond and thyme tart
34, 35
Tenderstem broccoli, feta,
muhammara and charred broccoli
ciabatta sandwiches 42, *43*
toast
cured salmon avocado toast 160
French onion soup with goats'
cheese toasts 64
fried courgettes on toast with ricotta
and fresh herbs 46, *47*
hummus toast with tomatoes,
chickpeas and crispy kale 120
tofu
coconut curry zoodles with Asian
greens and silken tofu 82, *83*
slow cooker ramen 85
spicy cucumber and silken tofu rice
noodles 148, *149*
sweet chilli and pepper barbecue
tofu skewers 116
Tex-Mex tofu scramble 124
tofu bánh mì sandwich 80, *81*
tomato 26, 65, 70, 88, 117, 126, 131–2,
138, 142, 163, 184, 211
baked gnocchi with tomatoes, basil
and marinated mozzarella 40, *41*
dukkah spaghetti with raw tomato
and almond sauce 136, *137*
flash-fried squid with chickpeas,
tomatoes and romesco 210
hummus toast with tomatoes,

chickpeas and crispy kale 120
pasta shells with fresh tomato, crab
and basil 188
roast aubergine and fresh tomato
salad with basil vinaigrette 118,
119
spinach and ricotta stuffed shells in
tomato sauce 50–2, *51–3*
tomato, almond and thyme tart
34, 35
tomato, basil and feta orzotto 38
tomato braised bean and white fish
stew with gremolata *176*, 177
tomato and chickpea alphabet
soup 66, 67
tomato and courgette baked eggs
36
tomato and root veggie casserole
with herby dumplings 9, 96–8, *97*
tomato salad with pomegranate
molasses 121
tomato (sun-dried) 117, 213
tomato, black olive and courgette
bread with anchovy butter 170–1,
171
tortilla 128
slow cooker spicy tortilla soup *130*,
131
tuna
Korean sashimi salad (*hwe dup
bap*) 156
ultimate tuna pasta 172, *173*

V

vinaigrette, basil vinaigrette 118, *119*

W

walnut 42, 107, 133
watermelon
vegan watermelon poke bowls
114, 115
watermelon, avocado and feta
salad with lime dressing 68, *69*
whitebait, fried whitebait sandwich
198, *199*

Acknowledgements

The list of people I want to thank is endless because this book really was a team effort from inception to print. No one involved in bringing these words, recipes, designs and photographs to life deserves to be left out, so if I have forgotten anyone, I'm sorry!

Diana, you are a wonderful literary agent and I honestly could not or would not want anyone better fighting my corner. Not only have you managed (again!) to get someone to publish my book, you're always there whenever I need someone to be my champion, my sounding board, and a much needed voice of sanity.

To the team at Yellow Kite and at Hodder. Thank you so much for asking me to write this book. It has honestly been one of the best experiences of my career so far with a couple of 'pinch me' moments thrown in for good measure! Lauren, I've loved having you as my editor – I hope that I've already thanked you enough for making sure I have been involved in every single step of the creative process. You recognised from our very first meeting how important this was to me. Amy, you've kept the trains running, put up with all my questions, helped me stick to deadlines and have generally been an all-round rockstar. Also thank you to everyone else who has worked on the text - especially my copy-editor Clare - and both the marketing and publicity teams.

Liz and Max, I still can't get over how beautiful all of the photos in this book are, especially the cover. I had no idea my recipes could look as good as they do in your photographs; I can't thank you enough. You guys set the tone for eight brilliant days in the studio which I think were the most fun I've ever had at 'work'. Charlie, thank you for hunting high and low to find the perfect backdrops, plates and pans, you helped make these beautiful photos happen. Nikki, I love everything about how the book looks, and that is down to you and your wonderful, fresh, modern design. Thank you also for your infectious energy every single day you were in the studio with us. Octavia, you were my hero. You helped make all the food look amazing, kept me company in the kitchen and taught me so much. My own pictures are already so much better thanks to everything I learnt from all of you on the shoot. Also, a special thank you to Lara for that extra day of help.

It almost goes without saying that I also need to thank my friends and my family. Thank you to everyone who was there to help and support me every step of the way. *One Pan Pescatarian* was all-consuming, and you all got me through it! Sherin, Martin, thank you for being my star recipe testers. You two are exactly the sort of people I wanted to write this book for, so having your input was invaluable! Daddy, Womble, yet again you let me take over your kitchen, lunch and dinner plans every time I came to visit. I know you're used to it by now, but I don't think I have thanked you enough.

J - I told you this book would take over our lives. Thank you, thank you, thank you for letting me feed you almost every single dish in this book for months on end. This book literally would not exist if you had not let that happen.

Finally, I want to thank to everyone who reads my blog each and every day. I'm lucky that I get to get up every morning, step into the kitchen and spend my day doing something I love. None of this would have been possible without you.

About the author

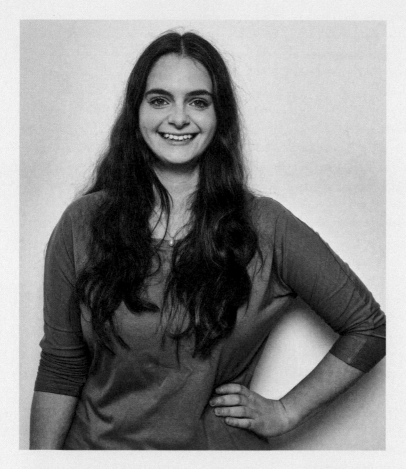

Rachel Phipps is a freelance food writer and recipe developer. She has written for *BBC Food*, *Refinery 29*, *Sainsbury's Magazine*, *The Times* and *Food 52*. She writes a popular food blog that celebrates the power of tasty, simple ideas to inspire weeknight cooking.